AF581770

Carborane: Dedicated to the Work of Professor Alan Welch

Carborane: Dedicated to the Work of Professor Alan Welch

Editors

Marina Yu. Stogniy
Georgina Rosair

MDPI • Basel • Beijing • Wuhan • Barcelona • Belgrade • Manchester • Tokyo • Cluj • Tianjin

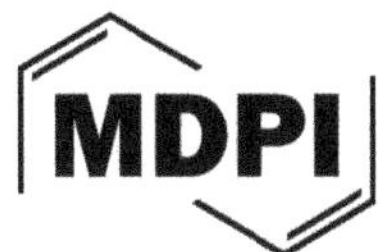

Editors
Marina Yu. Stogniy
A.N.Nesmeyanov Institute of Organoelement Compounds
of Russian Academy of Sciences
Moscow
Russia

Georgina Rosair
Heriot Watt University
Edinburgh
UK

Editorial Office
MDPI
St. Alban-Anlage 66
4052 Basel, Switzerland

This is a reprint of articles from the Special Issue published online in the open access journal *Crystals* (ISSN 2073-4352) (available at: https://www.mdpi.com/journal/crystals/special_issues/Carborane).

For citation purposes, cite each article independently as indicated on the article page online and as indicated below:

LastName, A.A.; LastName, B.B.; LastName, C.C. Article Title. *Journal Name* **Year**, *Volume Number*, Page Range.

ISBN 978-3-0365-3619-4 (Hbk)
ISBN 978-3-0365-3620-0 (PDF)

Contents

About the Editors

Marina Yu. Stogniy was born in Kazakhstan. In 2003-2009 she studied at the M.V. Lomonosov Moscow Institute of Fine Chemical Technology. She received her PhD degree in chemistry in 2013 under the supervision of Dr. Igor Sivaev. Dr Stogniy currently works as a Senior Researcher at the A.N. Nesmeyanov Institute of Organoelement Compounds of Russian Academy of Sciences (Laboratory of Organoaluminum and Organoboron Compounds) and teaches a course in general and inorganic chemistry at MIREA - Russian Technological University. Her areas of interest are the chemistry of polyhedral boron hydrides and metallocarboranes.

Georgina Rosair was born in Essex, England. She studied chemistry at Bristol University, obtaining a BSc in 1989, MSc in Analytical Chemistry in 1990 and a PhD in X-ray crystallography and computational chemistry with Prof Guy Orpen in 1994. In 1994 she became a postdoctoral worker in Prof. Alan Welch's group at Heriot Watt University, Edinburgh, to determine single crystal structures of carboranes and metallacarboranes, as well as crystal structure determinations for other research groups at Heriot Watt. In 1997 she became the staff crystallographer at Heriot Watt, the role expanded into powder diffraction and teaching inorganic chemistry, particularly practical laboratory courses. Since Prof Welch's retirement, her structure determination work now involves organometallic catalysts, supramolecular chemistry and organic photocatalysts and photosensitisers.

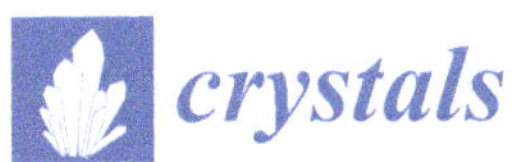 MDPI

Editorial

Carborane: Dedicated to the Work of Professor Alan Welch

Georgina M. Rosair [1,*] and Marina Yu. Stogniy [2,*]

1 Institute of Chemical Sciences, School of Engineering & Physical Sciences, Heriot Watt University, Edinburgh EH14 4AS, UK
2 A.N. Nesmeyanov Institute of Organoelement Compounds of Russian Academy of Sciences, 119991 Moscow, Russia
* Correspondence: g.m.rosair@hw.ac.uk (G.M.R.); stogniymarina@rambler.ru (M.Y.S.)

In the 1950s, borohydrides arose as promising components of new rocket and aviation fuels. This led to the discovery of a new class of compounds—polyhedral boron hydrides and the creation of a new chapter in the chemistry of organoelement compounds, which are intrinsically attractive structures. It was one of the most important discoveries of the 20th century in the field of chemistry.

Polyhedral boron hydrides lie at the intersection of organic and inorganic chemistry. The main theoretical interest in the chemistry of these compounds is due to their unusual type of chemical bond and their three-dimensional aromaticity. The aromatic nature of polyhedral boron hydrides determines many properties that distinguish them from most boron hydrides and organoboron compounds: high thermal stability, kinetic stability of the borane cluster, a pronounced tendency towards substitution reactions and isomerisations.

The replacement of one or more boron atoms in a polyhedral cluster by atoms of other elements enables further diversification. The formation of carboranes, i.e., the inclusion of one or two carbon atoms in a boron cluster, leads to some radical changes. On one hand, it is the acidic character of the CH protons that makes it possible to replace the hydrogen atom(s) with various functional groups using standard organic synthesis methods. On the other hand, it becomes possible to remove one or more boron vertices, which significantly expands the range of structural types of carboranes. Thus, in addition to closed (*closo*-carboranes) structures, open (*arachno*- and *nido*-carboranes) ones become accessible. Moreover, open structures, such as the 7,8-dicarba-*nido*-undecaborate anion (*nido*-carborane) and its derivatives, are very promising ligands for the synthesis of metal complexes. The deprotonated form of *nido*-carborane (dicarbollide dianion $[7,8\text{-}C_2B_9H_{11}]^{2-}$) is a three-dimensional cluster with an open pentagonal face capable of forming strong π-bonds with transition metal cations, which makes it a unique ligand with unusual steric, electronic and chemical properties that are sometimes inaccessible for organic ligands.

For more than half a century, scientists from all over the world have been studying the properties of carboranes, as well as the possibility of obtaining new substances and materials with desired properties. The study of these compounds significantly expanded the modern understanding of molecular structures and the nature of chemical bonds, such as Wade–Mingos rules and the three-dimensional aromaticity concept, which is currently used to describe the structure of not only polyhedral boron hydrides but also transition metal clusters, fullerenes and their derivatives, etc.

One of the scientists who made a significant contribution to the development of the chemistry of carboranes is the British chemist Alan Welch.

Alan Welch undertook his PhD with Mike Hursthouse (who established the National Crystallography Service in the UK), then a postdoctoral degree in heteroboranes with FGA Stone in Bristol, and another postdoctoral degree with H-B Bürgi at ETH Zürich. From a lectureship at Edinburgh University, he joined Heriot Watt University in 1994 and

Citation: Rosair, G.M.; Stogniy, M.Y. Carborane: Dedicated to the Work of Professor Alan Welch. *Crystals* **2021**, *11*, 1365. https://doi.org/10.3390/cryst11111365

Received: 4 November 2021
Accepted: 4 November 2021
Published: 9 November 2021

Publisher's Note: MDPI stays neutral with regard to jurisdictional claims in published maps and institutional affiliations.

established the crystallography facility at Heriot Watt, as well as leading his internationally recognized research group in heteroborane chemistry.

Later, Alan Welch worked on the synthesis of new heteroborane compounds, in particular, metallacarboranes. His group investigated their spectroscopic and structural characterization and studied their isomerisations and reactivity. The chemistry of supraicosahedral heteroboranes, bis(carboranes), nitrosocarboranes, and non-Wadian metallacarboranes was significantly expanded by Prof. Alan Welch's group.

These eight papers form a Special Issue of *Crystals* to commemorate the excellent contribution made to carborane chemistry by Prof. Alan Welch, who retired from Heriot Watt University, Edinburgh, this year.

The papers illustrate the very comprehensive world of heteroborane chemistry, from liquid crystals to BNCT agents, di-halogen bonding to quantum chemical calculations of tetrel complexes of the carbonium ylide $CB_{11}H_{11}$, nickellacarboranes as potential acid-base sensors to revealing how the selective formations of metallacarborane diastereomers can arise and metallacarboranes as radical cation salts with dielectric or semiconductor properties.

A computational study by Drahomír Hnyk and co-workers used DFT to successfully describe the reactions of experimentally known *closo*-$C_2B_8H_{10}$ with bases such as hydroxides and amines. The formation of [*arachno*-4,5-$C_2B_6H_{11}]^-$ was established computationally when this was not demonstrable experimentally [1].

Laskova and co-workers developed BNCT (boron neutron capture therapy) agents that incorporate amino acids that are potentially taken up by malignant brain tumour cells. The recent synthesis and biological evaluation of *m*-carboranyl-cysteine as an agent for boron neutron capture therapy inspired the group to synthesize the analogue based on readily available 1-mercapto-*o*-carborane. The synthesis was optimised by using the "free of base" method [2].

Mandal was one of Alan Welch's PhD students, and his work is on bis(nickelation) of bis(o-carborane), which forms diastereoisomeric mixtures on metalation of the second carborane cage and additionally undergoes isomerisation. It was found that stereospecificity was influenced by intramolecular dihydrogen bonding, whereas a specific isomerisation outcome was related to the stereo-electronic nature of bis(phosphine) ligands [3].

Liquid crystals incorporating carboranes were explored by Núñez and co-workers. They varied substituents on *o*-carborane to tune liquid crystal properties employing the mesogen cholesteryl benzoate. They found that the methyl substituent produced a blue phase, whilst the phenyl substituent species was not mesogenic [4].

Stogniy, Sivaev and co-workers synthesized half-sandwich nickel(II) complexes with amidine ligands where breakage of the Ni–N bond on acidification results in a colour change, which gives these complexes potential as acid-base indicators [5].

High-level quantum-chemical computations (G4MP2) were employed by Oliva-Enrich and co-workers to examine tetrel bonding (interaction between any electron donating system and a group of 14 elements acting as a Lewis acid) to predict the formation of tetrel complexes between the icosahedral carbonium ylide $CB_{11}H_{11}$ and a set of simple molecules and anions. The electronic structure of the complexes was analysed with AIM and ELF methods, showing the C--- X sharing and closed-shell interactions in the complexes [6].

Intermolecular halogen bonding, in this case, the diiodo bond, was investigated by Sivaev and co-workers. They obtained 1,12-diiodo-*ortho*-carborane, and its crystal structure was determined by X-ray diffraction, which revealed the existence of the I--- I halogen bond in its crystal structure. Such dihalogen bonding is not found in 1,12-dibromo-*ortho*-carborane. Quantum chemical calculations determined the noncovalent interaction preferences in 1,12-diiodo- and 1,12-dibromo-*ortho*-carboranes, which were in agreement with experimental findings [7].

Radical-cation salts based on tetramethyltetrathiafulvalene (TMTTF) and tetramethyltetraselenefulvalene (TMsTSF) with metallacarborane anions were also explored by Sivaev and co-workers. The iron bis(1,2-dicarbollide) and chromium bis(1,2-dicarbollide) salts were synthesized by electrocrystallisation, and their characterisation revealed that the resulting TMTTF radical-cation salts are dielectrics, whilst the TMTSF species is a narrow-gap semiconductor [8].

Thus, this Special Issue combines the latest achievements in the field of theoretical and experimental chemistry of carboranes. We thank all the authors who took part in this issue and look forward to further fruitful and impressive developments in the chemistry of carboranes.

Conflicts of Interest: The authors declare no conflict of interest.

References

1. Holub, J.; Fanfrlík, J.; McKee, M.L.; Hnyk, D. Reactions of Experimentally Known *Closo*-$C_2B_8H_{10}$ with Bases: A Computational Study. *Crystals* **2020**, *10*, 896. [CrossRef]
2. Laskova, J.; Kosenko, I.; Ananyev, I.; Stogniy, M.; Sivaev, I.; Bregadze, V. "Free of Base" Sulfa-Michael Addition for Novel *o*-Carboranyl-DL-Cysteine Synthesis. *Crystals* **2020**, *10*, 1133. [CrossRef]
3. Mandal, D.; Rosair, G.M. Exploration of Bis(nickelation) of 1,1′-Bis(*o*-carborane). *Crystals* **2021**, *11*, 16. [CrossRef]
4. Ferrer-Ugalde, A.; González-Campo, A.; Planas, J.G.; Viñas, C.; Teixidor, F.; Sáez, I.M.; Núñez, R. Tuning the Liquid Crystallinity of Cholesteryl-*o*-Carborane Dyads: Synthesis, Structure, Photoluminescence, and Mesomorphic Properties. *Crystals* **2021**, *11*, 133. [CrossRef]
5. Stogniy, M.Y.; Erokhina, S.A.; Suponitsky, K.Y.; Sivaev, I.B.; Bregadze, V.I. Coordination Ability of 10-EtC(NHPr)=HN-7,8-$C_2B_9H_{11}$ in the Reactions with Nickel(II) Phosphine Complexes. *Crystals* **2021**, *11*, 306. [CrossRef]
6. Ferrer, M.; Alkorta, I.; Elguero, J.; Oliva-Enrich, J.M. Carboranes as Lewis Acids: Tetrel Bonding in $CB_{11}H_{11}$ Carbonium Ylide. *Crystals* **2021**, *11*, 391. [CrossRef]
7. Suponitsky, K.Y.; Anisimov, A.A.; Anufriev, S.A.; Sivaev, I.B.; Bregadze, V.I. 1,12-Diiodo-*Ortho*-Carborane: A Classic Textbook Example of the Dihalogen Bond. *Crystals* **2021**, *11*, 396. [CrossRef]
8. Chudak, D.M.; Kazheva, O.N.; Kosenko, I.D.; Shilov, G.V.; Sivaev, I.B.; Abashev, G.G.; Shklyaeva, E.V.; Buravov, L.I.; Pevtsov, D.N.; Starodub, T.N.; et al. New Radical-Cation Salts Based on the TMTTF and TMTSF Donors with Iron and Chromium Bis(Dicarbollide) Complexes: Synthesis, Structure, Properties. *Crystals* **2021**, *11*, 1118. [CrossRef]

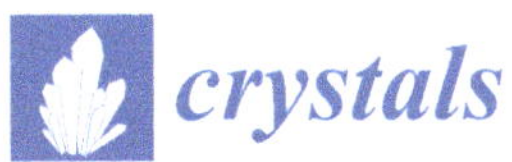 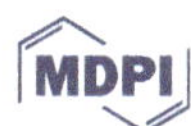

Communication

New Radical-Cation Salts Based on the TMTTF and TMTSF Donors with Iron and Chromium Bis(Dicarbollide) Complexes: Synthesis, Structure, Properties †

Denis M. Chudak [1], Olga N. Kazheva [2,3,*], Irina D. Kosenko [4], Gennady V. Shilov [2], Igor B. Sivaev [4,5], Georgy G. Abashev [6], Elena V. Shklyaeva [6], Lev I. Buravov [2], Dmitry N. Pevtsov [2], Tatiana N. Starodub [7], Vladimir I. Bregadze [4] and Oleg A. Dyachenko [2]

1 Chemistry Department, V. N. Karazin Kharkiv National University, 4 Svoboda Sq., 61077 Kharkiv, Ukraine; chudakdenis@gmail.com
2 Institute of Problems of Chemical Physics, Russian Academy of Sciences, 1 Semenov Av., 142432 Chernogolovka, Moscow Region, Russia; genshil@icp.ac.ru (G.V.S.); buravov@icp.ac.ru (L.I.B.); pevtsovdm@gmail.com (D.N.P.); doa@rfbr.ru (O.A.D.)
3 Institute of Experimental Mineralogy, Russian Academy of Sciences, 4 Academician Osypyan Str., 4, 142432 Chernogolovka, Moscow Region, Russia
4 A.N. Nesmeyanov Institute of Organoelement Compounds, Russian Academy of Sciences, 28 Vavilov Str., 119991 Moscow, Russia; kosenko@ineos.ac.ru (I.D.K.); sivaev@ineos.ac.ru (I.B.S.); bre@ineos.ac.ru (V.I.B.)
5 Basic Department of Chemistry of Innovative Materials and Technologies, G.V. Plekhanov Russian University of Economics, 36 Stremyannyi Line, 117997 Moscow, Russia
6 Organic Chemistry Department, Perm State University, 15 Bukirev Str., 614990 Perm, Russia; gabashev@psu.ru (G.G.A.); EV_Shklyaeva@psu.ru (E.V.S.)
7 Institute of Chemistry, Jan Kochanowski University, 15G Swietokrzyska Str., 25-406 Kielce, Poland; tstarodub@ujk.edu.pl
* Correspondence: koh@icp.ac.ru
† Dedicated to Professor Alan J. Welch in recognition of his outstanding contribution to the chemistry of carboranes.

Citation: Chudak, D.M.; Kazheva, O.N.; Kosenko, I.D.; Shilov, G.V.; Sivaev, I.B.; Abashev, G.G.; Shklyaeva, E.V.; Buravov, L.I.; Pevtsov, D.N.; Starodub, T.N.; et al. New Radical-Cation Salts Based on the TMTTF and TMTSF Donors with Iron and Chromium Bis(Dicarbollide) Complexes: Synthesis, Structure, Properties. *Crystals* **2021**, *11*, 1118. https://doi.org/10.3390/cryst11091118

Academic Editors: Georgina Rosair and Marina Yu. Stogniy

Received: 11 August 2021
Accepted: 9 September 2021
Published: 14 September 2021

Abstract: New radical-cation salts based on tetramethyltetrathiafulvalene (TMTTF) and tetramethyltetraselenefulvalene (TMsTSF) with metallacarborane anions (TMTTF)[3,3′-Cr(1,2-$C_2B_9H_{11})_2$], (TMTTF)[3,3′-Fe(1,2-$C_2B_9H_{11})_2$], and $(TMTSF)_2$[3,3′-Cr(1,2-$C_2B_9H_{11})_2$] were synthesized by electrocrystallization. Their crystal structures were determined by single crystal X-ray diffraction, and their electrophysical properties in a wide temperature range were studied. The first two salts are dielectrics, while the third one is a narrow-gap semiconductor: $\sigma_{RT} = 5 \times 10^{-3}$ $Ohm^{-1}cm^{-1}$; $E_a \approx 0.04$ eV (aprox. 320 cm^{-1}).

Keywords: iron bis(1,2-dicarbollide); chromium bis(1,2-dicarbollide); tetramethyltetrathiafulvalene; tetramethyltetraselenafulvalene; radical-cation salts; crystal and molecular structure; electric conductivity

1. Introduction

Radical-cation salts and charge transfer complexes based on derivatives of tetrathiafulvalene (TTF) constitute a wide class of organic materials with transport properties ranging from insulating to superconducting [1–4]. This work is part of the systematic study of radical-cation salts of tetrathiafulvalene and its derivatives with metallacarborane anions, of which earlier results were summarized in works [5–7].

Transition metal bis(dicarbollide) complexes [3,3′-M(1,2-$C_2B_9H_{11})_2]^-$ (M = Fe, Co, or Ni) are of great interest as counterions for the synthesis of TTF-based molecular conductors due to the unique high stability, possibility of tuning the charge and nature of the metal, and wide range of options for modification with dicarbollide ligands via hydrogen substitution by other atoms and functional groups [5,6]. Although most of the compounds studied were BEDT-TTF-based radical-cation salts, recently, we have synthesized radical-cation salts based on such unconventional and rather exotic donors as bis(1,3-propylenedithio)-tetrathiafulvalene [8,9], dibenzotetrathiafulvalene [10], and 4,5-ethylenedithio-4′,5′-(2-oxa-1,3-propylenedithio)-tetrathiafulvalene [9]. On the other hand, although compounds of the composition $(TMTXF)_2Y$ (X = T, S) are usually classical organic metals among which the first organic superconductors were discovered [4,7], and TMTTF and TMTSF radical-cation salts continue to attract the attention of researchers [11–15], very little attention has been paid to TMTTF and TMTSF radical-cation salts with metallacarborane anions [16–19]. This prompted us to prepare and investigate new TMTTF and TMTSF radical-cation salts with metallacarborane anions.

This contribution describes the synthesis, structure, and electrical conductivity of new salts with TMTTF and TMTSF radical-cations and metallacarborane anions: (TMTTF)[3,3′-Cr(1,2-$C_2B_9H_{11})_2$] (**1**), (TMTTF)[3,3′-Fe(1,2-$C_2B_9H_{11})_2$] (**2**), and $(TMTSF)_2$[3,3′- Cr(1,2-$C_2B_9H_{11})_2$] (**3**).

2. Results and Discussion

Single crystals of compounds **1–3** suitable for X-ray diffraction studies in the form of thin plates were obtained by electrochemical crystallization (See Supplementary Materials and Table 1). The crystal structure of **1** is formed by the TMTTF radical-cations and the [3,3′-Cr(1,2-$C_2B_9H_{11})_2]^-$ anions occupying general positions in the unit cell (Figure 1). (TMTTF)[3,3′-Cr(1,2-$C_2B_9H_{11})_2$] has a pseudo-layered structure, in which anionic layers alternate along the *ac* diagonal with layers formed by radical-cation dimers (Figure 2). The dimer formation corresponds to the stoichiometry of the salt: in this case due to the Peierls instability a phase transition should occur with doubling of the stacks period [7]. The distances between the averaged planes of the TMTTF donors in the dimers are 3.38 Å (the planes are drawn through all S atoms), and the dihedral angle between the planes is 0° by symmetry conditions. There are short intermolecular S . . . S interactions (3.426(1)–3.432(1) Å) of the "face-to-face" type between the TMTTF donors in the dimers.

Table 1. Crystal data and structure refinement for (TMTTF)[3,3′-Cr(1,2-$C_2B_9H_{11})_2$] (**1**), (TMTTF)[3,3′-Fe(1,2-$C_2B_9H_{11})_2$] (**2**), and $(TMTSF)_2$[3,3′-Cr(1,2-$C_2B_9H_{11})_2$] (**3**).

Compound	(1)	(2)	(3)
Empiric formula	$C_{14}H_{34}B_{18}CrS_4$	$C_{14}H_{34}B_{18}FeS_4$	$C_{24}H_{46}B_{18}CrSe_8$
Formula weight	577.23	581.08	1212.87
Crystal system	Monoclinic	Monoclinic	Triclinic
Space group	$P2_1/c$	$C2/m$	$P\,1$
a (Å)	11.726(2)	17.3487(8)	7.451(4)
b (Å)	12.753(2)	12.0235(6)	12.342(6)
c (Å)	19.387(3)	6.6791(3)	12.961(7)
α (°)	90	90	117.743(7)
β (°)	102.701(2)	90.7840(6)	92.344(8)
γ (°)	90	90	100.325(8)
V (Å^3)	2828.3(6)	1393.08(11)	1027.1(9)
Z	4	2	1
λ (Å)	0.71073	0.71073	0.71073
D_{calc} (Mg m^{-3})	1.36	1.38	1.96
μ (mm^{-1})	0.708	0.850	7.388
Number of reflections collected	28470	11191	4513
Number of independent reflections	8147	2319	4513
Number of reflections with $[F_0 > 4\sigma(F_0)]$	6787	2183	3754
Number of parameters refined	426	130	233
$(2\theta)_{max}$ (°)	60.48	63.70	55.44
R	0.037	0.021	0.051

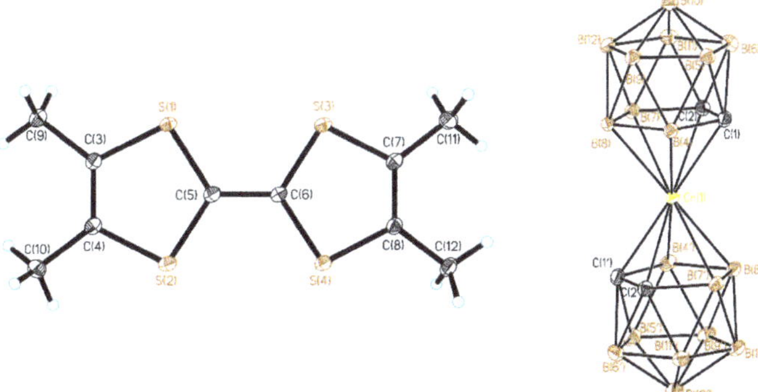

Figure 1. TMTTF radical-cation and anion in (**1**). Thermal ellipsoids are given at 30% probability level. Cage H atoms omitted for clarity.

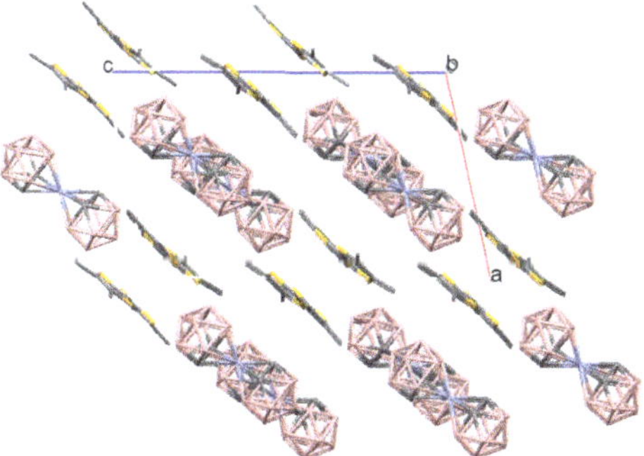

Figure 2. Crystal packing fragment of (**1**). A view along the *b* axis. The unit cell is outlined. H atoms are omitted for clarity.

The $TMTTF^+$ radical-cations are non-planar and have a "boat" conformation: the maximum deviations of terminal C(9), C(10), C(11), and C(12) atoms from the plane of the averaged molecule drawn through all sulfur atoms are 0.30–0.36 Å.

The Cr-C and Cr-B bond lengths are 2.173(2)–2.180(2) and 2.232(2)–2.279(2) Å, correspondingly. The distances from the chromium atom to the C_2B_3 faces of the dicarbollide ligands are equal to 1.68 Å, which is close to the corresponding distances found in the structures of Cs $[3,3'\text{-}Cr(1,2\text{-}C_2B_9H_{11})_2]$ [20], (TTF)$[3,3'\text{-}Cr(1,2\text{-}C_2B_9H_{11})_2]$ [21], and (BEDT-TTF)$_2[3,3'\text{-}Cr(1,2\text{-}C_2B_9H_{11})_2]$ [22,23]. The dicarbollide ligands in the $[3,3'\text{-}Cr(1,2\text{-}C_2B_9H_{11})_2]^-$ anion are turned relative to each other by 180°, forming the *transoid* conformation. The C_2B_3 faces deviate slightly from parallel, being inclined by 178.7° to each other.

The electrical conductivity measurements have shown that 1 is an insulator with $\sigma_{293}{\sim}10^{-11}$ Ohm^{-1}cm^{-1}. The low value of electrical conductivity is apparently connected with the absence of conducting layers and dimerization of the radical-cations stacks.

It should be noted that compound 1 is the first TMTTF radical-cation salt with an unsubstituted transition metal bis(dicarbollide), while the radical-cation salts (TMTTF)$[8\text{-}HO\text{-}3,3'\text{-}Co(1,2\text{-}C_2B_9H_{10})(1',2'\text{-}C_2B_9H_{11})]$ and (TMTTF)$(8,8'\text{-}Cl_2\text{-}3,3'\text{-}Co(1,2\text{-}C_2B_9H_{10})_2]_2$ obtained earlier contained substituted bis(dicarbollide) anions [16,17].

The crystal structure of (TMTTF)$[3,3'\text{-}Fe(1,2\text{-}C_2B_9H_{11})_2]$ (**2**) is formed by a quarter of the TMTTF radical-cation in a special position placed on the *m* plane and a quarter of the $[3,3'\text{-}Fe(1,2\text{-}C_2B_9H_{11})_2]^-$ anion in the *2/m* special position of the unit cell (Figure 3). The compound **2** is characterized by a structure where the TMTTF cations and the metallacarborane anions form staggered stacks (Figures 4 and 5). The distances between the averaged planes of the TMTTF donors in the dimers are 3.38 Å, and the dihedral angle between the planes is 0° by symmetry conditions.

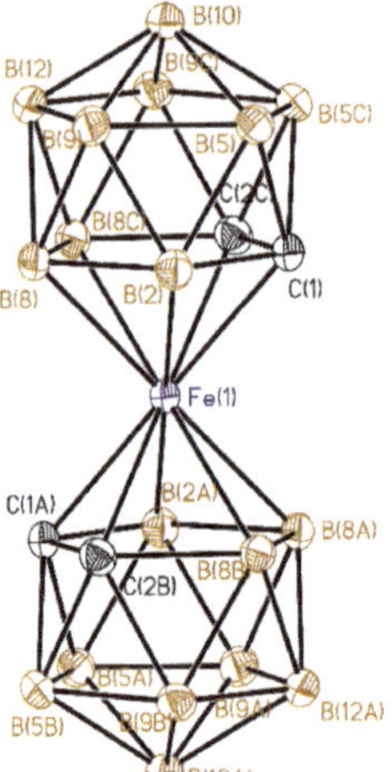

Figure 3. Anion in (**2**). Thermal ellipsoids are given at 30% probability level. Cage H atoms omitted for clarity.

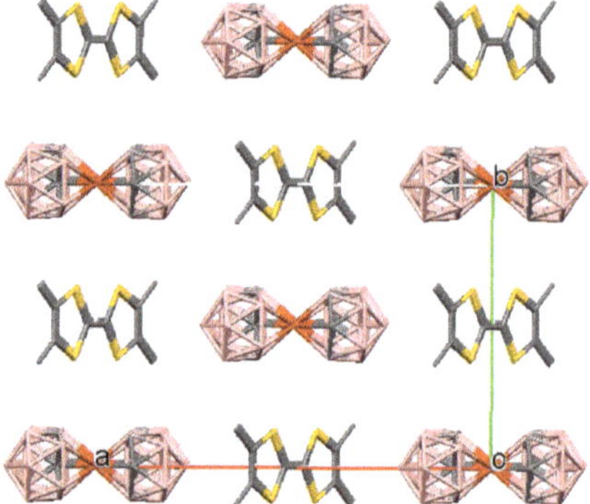

Figure 4. Crystal packing fragment of (**2**). A view along the *c* axis. The unit cell is outlined. H atoms are omitted for clarity.

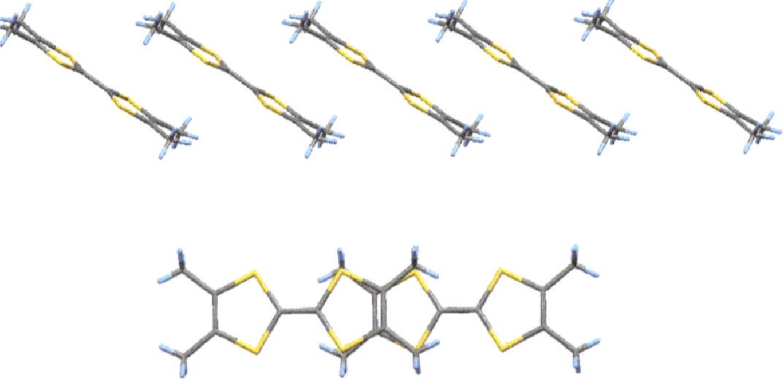

Figure 5. A stack and radical-cations overlapping in (**2**).

The Fe-C and Fe-B bond lengths are 2.0790(9)–2.1001(8) and 2.1001(8)–2.1494(8) Å, correspondingly, and the overlapping values are due to the statistical disordering of carbon and boron atoms in the dicarbollide ligands. The distances from the iron atom to the C_2B_3 faces of the dicarbollide ligands are equal to 1.53 Å, which is close to the distances in analogous salts of the iron bis(dicarbollide) anion [19,24,25]. The dicarbollide ligands are turned relative to each by 180°, forming the *transoid* conformation. The C_2B_3 faces are parallel by symmetry conditions.

According to the electric conductivity measurements, compound 2 is an insulator with conductivity ~10^{-10} $Ohm^{-1}cm^{-1}$. The low value of electroconductivity is in an agreement with the 1:1 stoichiometry and non-layered structure of the salt, as well as with the inclination angle of the radical-cations in the stack, at which there is only slight overlap between neighboring radical-cations.

The $(TMTSF)_2[3,3'\text{-}Cr(1,2\text{-}C_2B_9H_{10})_2]$ (3) crystals are isostructural to $(TMTSF)_2[3,3'\text{-}Co(1,2\text{-}C_2B_9H_{11})_2]$ and $(TMTSF)_2[3,3'\text{-}Fe(1,2\text{-}C_2B_9H_{11})_2]$ salts studied earlier, containing cobalt and iron bis(dicarbollide) anions [18,19]. The crystal structure of 3 is formed by the TMTSF cation in a general position and the $[3,3'\text{-}Cr(1,2\text{-}C_2B_9H_{11})_2]^-$ anion in a special centrosymmetrical position (Figure 6). Compound 3 possesses a structure (Figures 7 and 8) where the $TMTSF^{+\bullet}$ radical-cations and anions form staggered stacks. The distances between the averaged planes of the TMTSF donors in the dimers are 3.70 and 3.73 Å, and the dihedral angle between the planes is 0° by symmetry conditions.

The Cr-C and Cr-B bond lengths are 2.175(7)–2.176(7) and 2.226(8)–2.277(8) Å, correspondingly. The distances from the chromium atom to the C_2B_3 faces of the dicarbollide ligands are equal to 1.68 Å, and the dicarbollide ligands in the $[3,3'\text{-}Cr(1,2\text{-}C_2B_9H_{10})_2]^-$ anion are turned relative to each other by 180°, forming the *transoid* conformation. The C_2B_3 faces are parallel to each other by the symmetry conditions.

The electroconductivity measurements have revealed that compound 3 in the range of 41–195 K behaves like a dielectric. However, above 195 K, the delocalization of the positive charge disappears due to the numerous intermolecular S . . . S contacts and an inconspicuous dielectric–semiconductor structural phase transition occurs, caused by charge ordering: stacks contain both TMTSF molecules and TMTSF radical-cations. The room temperature electric conductivity $\sigma_{293} = 5 \cdot 10^{-3}$ $Ohm^{-1}cm^{-1}$ and activation energy $E_a \cong 0.04$ eV (Figure 9). It should be noted that analogous salts $(TMTSF)_2[3,3'\text{-}Co(1,2\text{-}C_2B_9H_{11})_2]$ and $(TMTSF)_2[3,3'\text{-}Fe(1,2\text{-}C_2B_9H_{11})_2]$ were characterized by electroconductivity values σ_{293} of 15 and 0.1 $Ohm^{-1}cm^{-1}$, correspondingly [18,19].

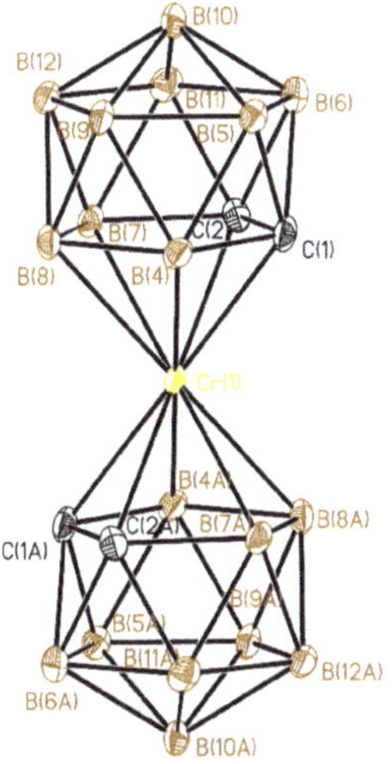

Figure 6. Anion in (**3**). Thermal ellipsoids are given at 30% probability level.

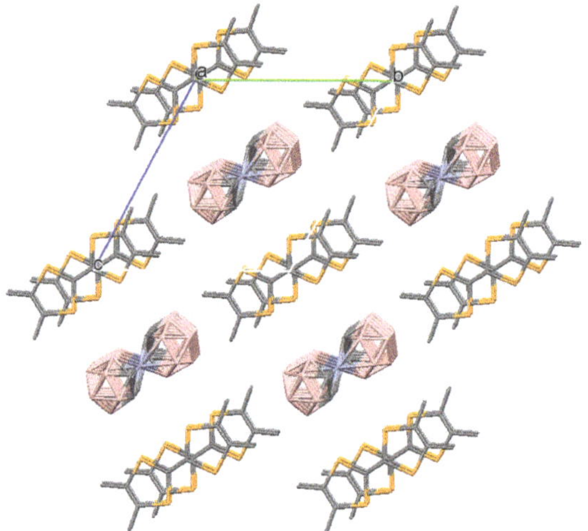

Figure 7. Crystal packing fragment of (**3**). A view along the *a* axis. The unit cell is outlined. H atoms are omitted for clarity.

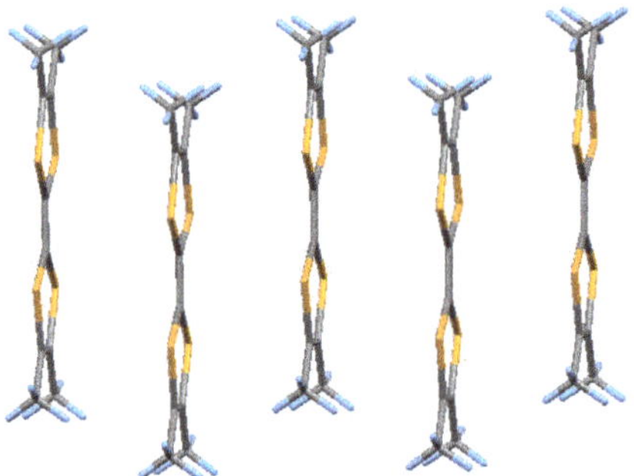

Figure 8. A stack of radical-cations in (**3**).

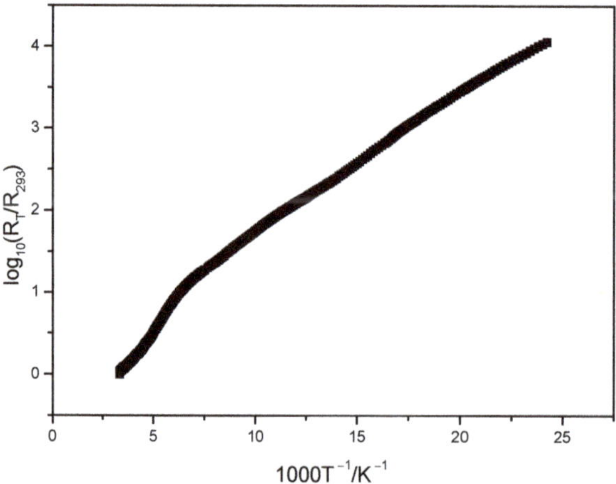

Figure 9. Temperature dependence of electrical resistivity of (**3**).

In conclusion, new salts with the TMTTF and TMTSF radical-cations and metallacarborane anions (TMTTF)[3,3′-Cr(1,2-$C_2B_9H_{11}$)$_2$] (**1**), (TMTTF)[3,3′-Fe(1,2-$C_2B_9H_{11}$)$_2$] (**2**), and $(TMTSF)_2$[3,3′-Cr(1,2-$C_2B_9H_{11}$)$_2$] (**3**) were electrochemically synthesized and investigated. Their crystal structures were determined by X-ray study and electroconductivities were measured. Salts (**1**) and (**2**) are insulators, which is explained by the 1:1 stoichiometry and the absence of an extended network of interdonor interactions, whereas (**3**) is a semiconductor at room temperature with electroconductivity $\sigma_{293} = 5 \cdot 10^{-3}$ $Ohm^{-1}cm^{-1}$, which is lower than in $(TMTSF)_2$[3,3′-Fe(1,2-$C_2B_9H_{11}$)$_2$] and $(TMTSF)_2$[3,3′-Co(1,2-$C_2B_9H_{11}$)$_2$] salts (electroconductivity values σ_{293} of 0.1 and 15 $Ohm^{-1}cm^{-1}$, correspondingly). The tendency of a rise in conductivity ($5 \cdot 10^{-3} < 0.1 < 15$) is apparently connected with decreasing the cation size in the order $Cr^{3+} > Fe^{3+} > Co^{3+}$ [26], which leads to decreasing the corresponding metallacarborane anion size and, in turn, to unit cell compression and a tighter radical-cation packing of the salts.

Supplementary Materials: Details of experimental data including synthesis of the title compounds, their X-ray diffraction studies, and electric resistivity measurements are available online at https://www.mdpi.com/article/10.3390/cryst11091118/s1.

Author Contributions: Synthesis, D.M.C., I.B.S., I.D.K., G.G.A., E.V.S.; measurements, L.I.B., D.N.P., T.N.S.; X-ray diffraction study, G.V.S.; data analysis and writing, O.N.K.; research conception, V.I.B., O.A.D. All authors have read and agreed to the published version of the manuscript.

Funding: This research received no external funding.

Institutional Review Board Statement: Not applicable.

Informed Consent Statement: Not applicable.

Data Availability Statement: The crystallographic data for this paper (the CCDC numbers 2091714, 2091713, 2091715 for (**1**), (**2**), (**3**), respectively) can be obtained free of charge via www.ccdc.cam.ac.uk/data_request/cif (accessed on 11 August 2021).

Acknowledgments: This work was partly performed in accordance with the state task of the Institute of Problems of Chemical Physics, Russian Academy of Sciences, State Registration No. AAAA-A19-119092390076-7. Synthesis and characterization of the starting metallacarboranes were performed at A.N. Nesmeyanov Institute of Organoelement Compounds, Russian Academy of Sciences with support of the Ministry of Science and Higher Education of the Russian Federation.

Conflicts of Interest: The authors declare no conflict of interest. The funders had no role in the design of the study; in the collection, analyses, or interpretation of data; in the writing of the manuscript, or in the decision to publish the results.

References

1. Williams, J.M.; Ferraro, J.R.; Thorn, R.J.; Carlson, K.D.; Geiser, U.; Wang, H.H.; Kini, A.M.; Whangbo, M.-H. *Organic SuperConductors (Including Fullerenes: Synthesis, Structure, Properties, and Theory)*; Prentice Hall: Englewood Cliffs, NJ, USA, 1992.
2. Ishiguro, T.; Yamaji, K.; Saito, G. *Organic Superconductors*, 2nd ed.; Springer Series in Solid-State Sciences; Springer: Berlin, Germany, 1998.
3. Saito, G.; Yoshida, Y. Organic superconductors. *Chem. Rec.* **2011**, *11*, 124–145. [CrossRef]
4. Naito, T. Modern history of organic conductors: An overview. *Crystals* **2021**, *11*, 838. [CrossRef]
5. Bregadze, V.I.; Dyachenko, O.A.; Kazheva, O.N.; Kravchenko, A.V.; Sivaev, I.B.; Starodub, V.A. Tetrathiafulvalene-based radical-cation salts with transition metal bis(dicarbollide) anions. *CrystEngComm* **2015**, *17*, 4754–4767. [CrossRef]
6. Bregadze, V.I.; Dyachenko, O.A.; Kazheva, O.N.; Kosenko, I.D.; Kravchenko, A.V.; Sivaev, I.B.; Starodub, V.A. Electroconducting radical-cation salts based on tetrathiafulvalene derivatives and transition metals bis(dicarbollides). *Russ. J. Gen. Chem.* **2019**, *89*, 971–987. [CrossRef]
7. Starodub, V.A.; Starodub, T.N.; Kazheva, O.N.; Bregadze, V.I. *Materialy Sovremennoi Electroniki i Spintroniki (Materials of Modern Electronics and Spintronics)*; Fizmatlit: Moscow, Russia, 2018; 424p.
8. Kazheva, O.N.; Chudak, D.M.; Shilov, G.V.; Komissarova, E.A.; Kosenko, I.D.; Kravchenko, A.V.; Shilova, I.A.; Shklyaeva, E.V.; Abashev, G.G.; Sivaev, I.B.; et al. First molecular conductors of BPDT-TTF with metallacarborane anions: (BPDT-TTF)[3,3′-Cr(1,2-$C_2B_9H_{11}$)$_2$] and (BPDT-TTF)[3,3′-Co(1,2-$C_2B_9H_{11}$)$_2$]—Synthesis, structure, properties. *J. Organomet. Chem.* **2018**, *867*, 375–380. [CrossRef]

9. Kazheva, O.N.; Chudak, D.M.; Shilov, G.V.; Kosenko, I.D.; Abashev, G.G.; Shklyaeva, E.V.; Kravchenko, A.V.; Starodub, V.A.; Buravov, L.I.; Dyachenko, O.A.; et al. First EOTT and BPDT-TTF based molecular conductors with $[8,8'-Cl_2-3,3'-Fe(1,2-C_2B_9H_{10})_2]^-$ anion—Synthesis, structure, properties. *J. Organomet. Chem.* **2021**, *949*, 121956. [CrossRef]
10. Kazheva, O.N.; Chudak, D.M.; Shilov, G.V.; Kravchenko, A.V.; Kosenko, I.D.; Sivaev, I.B.; Abashev, G.G.; Shklyaeva, E.V.; Starodub, V.A.; Buravov, L.I.; et al. First radical-cation salts based on dibenzotetrathiafulvalene (DBTTF) with metallacarborane anions: Synthesis, structure, properties. *J. Organomet. Chem.* **2020**, *930*, 121592. [CrossRef]
11. Mroweh, N.; Mézière, C.; Allain, M.; Auban-Senzier, P.; Canadell, E.; Avarvari, N. Conservation of structural arrangements and 3:1 stoichiometry in a series of crystalline conductors of TMTTF, TMTSF, BEDT-TTF, and chiral DM-EDT-TTF with the oxo-bis[pentafluorotantalate(V)] dianion. *Chem. Sci.* **2020**, *11*, 10078–10091. [CrossRef] [PubMed]
12. Yoshino, H.; Iwasaki, Y.; Tanaka, R.; Tsujimoto, Y.; Matsuoka, C. Crystal structures and electrical resistivity of three exotic TMTSF salts with I_3^-: Determination of valence by DFT and MP2 calculations. *Crystals* **2020**, *10*, 1119. [CrossRef]
13. Sahadevan, S.A.; Abhervé, A.; Monni, N.; Auban-Senzier, P.; Cui, H.; Kato, R.; Mercuri, M.L.; Avarvari, N. Radical-cation salts of tetramethyltetrathiafulvalene (TM-TTF) and tetramethyltetraselenafulvalene (TM-TSF) with chlorocyananilate-based anions. *Cryst. Growth Des.* **2020**, *20*, 6777–6786. [CrossRef]
14. Frąckowiak, A.; Barszcz, B.; Olejniczak, I.; Tomasik, M.; Jarzyniak, N.; Świetlik, R.; Auban-Senzier, P.; Fourmigué, M.; Jeannin, O.; Camerel, F. Mixed valence trimers in cation radical salts of TMTTF with the planar bis(6-sulfo-8-quinolato) platinum complex $[Pt(qS)_2]^{2-}$. *New J. Chem.* **2020**, *44*, 15538–15548. [CrossRef]
15. Allain, M.; Mézière, C.; Auban-Senzier, P.; Avarvari, N. Old donors for new molecular conductors: Combining TMTSF and BEDT-TTF with anionic $(TaF_6)_{1-x}/(PF_6)_x$ alloys. *Crystals* **2021**, *11*, 386. [CrossRef]
16. Kazheva, O.N.; Alexandrov, G.G.; Kravchenko, A.V.; Kosenko, I.D.; Lobanova, I.A.; Sivaev, I.B.; Filippov, O.A.; Shubina, E.S.; Bregadze, V.I.; Starodub, V.A.; et al. Molecular conductors with a 8-hydroxy cobalt bis(dicarbollide) anion. *Inorg. Chem.* **2011**, *50*, 444–450. [CrossRef] [PubMed]
17. Kazheva, O.N.; Alexandrov, G.G.; Kravchenko, A.V.; Sivaev, I.B.; Starodub, V.A.; Kosenko, I.D.; Lobanova, I.A.; Bregadze, V.I.; Buravov, L.I.; Dyachenko, O.A. New organic conductors with halogen and phenyl substituted cobalt bis(dicarbollide) anions. *J. Chem. Eng. Chem. Res.* **2015**, *2*, 497–503.
18. Kazheva, O.N.; Chekhlov, A.N.; Alexandrov, G.G.; Buravov, L.I.; Kravchenko, A.V.; Starodub, V.A.; Sivaev, I.B.; Bregadze, V.I.; Dyachenko, O.A. Synthesis, structure and electrical conductivity of fulvalenium salts of cobalt bis(dicarbollide) anion. *J. Organomet. Chem.* **2006**, *691*, 4225–4233. [CrossRef]
19. Kazheva, O.N.; Alexandrov, G.G.; Kravchenko, A.V.; Starodub, V.A.; Sivaev, I.B.; Lobanova, I.A.; Bregadze, V.I.; Buravov, L.I.; Dyachenko, O.A. New fulvalenium salts of bis(dicarbollide) cobalt and iron: Synthesis, crystal structure and electrical conductivity. *J. Organomet. Chem.* **2007**, *692*, 5033–5043. [CrossRef]
20. Bednarska-Szczepaniak, K.; Przelazły, E.; Kania, K.D.; Szwed, M.; Litecká, M.; Grüner, B.; Leśnikowski, Z.J. Interaction of adenosine, modified using carborane clusters, with ovarian cancer cells: A new anticancer approach against chemoresistance. *Cancers* **2021**, *13*, 3855. [CrossRef] [PubMed]
21. Forward, J.M.; Mingos, D.M.P.; Müller, T.E.; Williams, D.J.; Yan, Y.-K. Synthesis and structural characterization of metallacarborane sandwich salts with tetrathiafulvalene (ttf) $[M(C_2B_9H_{11})_2][ttf]$ (M = Cr, Fe, Ni). *J. Organomet. Chem.* **1994**, *467*, 207–216. [CrossRef]
22. Yan, Y.-K.; Mingos, D.M.P.; Williams, D.J.; Kurmoo, M. Synthesis, structures and physical properties of bis(ethylenedithio) tetrathiafulvalenium salts of paramagnetic metallacarborane anions. *J. Chem. Soc. Dalton Trans.* **1995**, *19*, 3221–3230. [CrossRef]
23. Čižmár, E.; Šoltésová, D.; Kazheva, O.N.; Alexandrov, G.G.; Kravchenko, A.V.; Chekulaeva, L.A.; Kosenko, I.D.; Sivaev, I.B.; Bregadze, V.I.; Fedorchenko, A.V.; et al. Large magnetic anisotropy of chromium(III) ions in a bis(ethylenedithio)tetrathiafulvalenium salt of chromium bis(dicarbollide), $(ET)_2[3,3'-Cr(1,2-C_2B_9H_{11})_2]$. *Trans. Met. Chem.* **2018**, *43*, 647–655. [CrossRef]
24. Sivaev, I.B.; Bregadze, V.I. Chemistry of nickel and iron bis(dicarbollides). *J. Organomet. Chem.* **2000**, *614–615*, 27–36. [CrossRef]
25. Kazheva, O.N.; Alexandrov, G.G.; Kravchenko, A.V.; Sivaev, I.B.; Kosenko, I.D.; Lobanova, I.A.; Kajňakov, M.; Buravov, L.I.; Bregadze, V.I.; Feher, A.; et al. Synthesis, structure, electrical and magnetic properties of $(BEDT-TTF)_2[3,3-Fe(1,2-C_2B_9H_{11})_2]$. *Inorg. Chem. Commun.* **2012**, *15*, 106–108. [CrossRef]
26. Shannon, R.D. Revised effective ionic radii and systematic studies of interatomic distances in halides and chalcogenides. *Acta Cryst. C* **1976**, *32*, 751–767. [CrossRef]

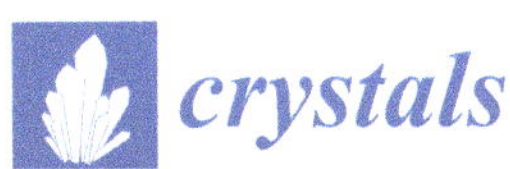 MDPI

Communication

1,12-Diiodo-*Ortho*-Carborane: A Classic Textbook Example of the Dihalogen Bond †

Kyrill Yu. Suponitsky [1,*], Alexei A. Anisimov [1,2], Sergey A. Anufriev [1], Igor B. Sivaev [1,*] and Vladimir I. Bregadze [1]

[1] A.N. Nesmeyanov Institute of Organoelement Compounds, Russian Academy of Sciences, 28 Vavilov Str., 119991 Moscow, Russia; anisimov.alex.a@gmail.com (A.A.A.); trueman476@mail.ru (S.A.A.); bre@ineos.ac.ru (V.I.B.)

[2] Higher Chemical College at the Russian Academy of Sciences, D.I. Mendeleev Russian Chemical Technological University, 9 Miusskaya Sq., 125047 Moscow, Russia

* Correspondence: kirshik@yahoo.com (K.Y.S.); sivaev@ineos.ac.ru (I.B.S.)

† Dedicated to Professor Alan J. Welch in occasion of his retirement at Herriot-Watt University and in recognition of his outstanding contribution in the carborane chemistry.

Abstract: The crystal structure of 1,12-diiodo-*ortho*-carborane 1,12-I_2-1,2-$C_2B_{10}H_{10}$ was determined by single crystal X-ray diffraction. In contrary to earlier studied 1,12-dibromo analogue 1,12-Br_2-1,2-$C_2B_{10}H_{10}$, its crystal packing is governed by the presence of the intermolecular I···I dihalogen bonds between the iodine atom attached to the carbon atom (acceptor) and the iodine atom attached to the antipodal boron atom (donor) of the carborane cage. The observed dihalogen bonds belong to the II type and are characterized by classical parameters: shortened I···I distance of 3.5687(9) Å, C–I···I angle of 172.61(11)° and B–I···I angle of 92.98(12)°.

Keywords: carborane; iodo derivatives; dihalogen bond; X-ray structure; quantum chemical calculationsy

Citation: Suponitsky, K.Y.; Anisimov, A.A.; Anufriev, S.A.; Sivaev, I.B.; Bregadze, V.I. 1,12-Diiodo-*Ortho*-Carborane: A Classic Textbook Example of the Dihalogen Bond. *Crystals* **2021**, *11*, 396. https://doi.org/10.3390/cryst11040396

Academic Editors: Georgina Rosair and Marina Yu. Stogniy

Received: 15 March 2021
Accepted: 6 April 2021
Published: 8 April 2021

1. Introduction

Carboranes $[CB_{11}H_{12}]^-$ and $C_2B_{10}H_{12}$, in which one or two vertices in boron icosahedron are replaced by a carbon unit, are a fascinating family of compounds with exceptional chemical and thermal robustness, unique geometry, rigidity, and synthetic versatility [1]. Selective chemical substitution of hydrogen atoms at carbon or boron atoms in these clusters allows for their use as rigid, three dimensional scaffolds upon which to construct new materials, such as liquid crystals [2–5], nonlinear optical materials [6–9], carborane-based anticrowns [10], and even in drug design [11,12]. As rigid molecules of fixed length, carboranes can be used as building blocks ("molecular tinkertoys") [13–18] for supramolecular assemblies, such as porous coordination polymers or metal–organic frameworks (MOFs) [19–22]. Another type of supramolecular structures with the participation of carboranes is based on the acidity of their CH groups, which demonstrate a high potential for hydrogen bonding. Indeed, intermolecular C–H···O and C–H···N hydrogen bonding, including bifurcated interactions, features in much of the supramolecular chemistry of carboranes [23,24]. Functionalization of carboranes with different substituents including halogen atoms opens an opportunity to the formation diverse noncovalent interactions [25,26]. Thus, the intermolecular C–H···X–B hydrogen bonds were found to stabilize crystal structures of fluoro- [27], bromo- [28] and iodo- [29–34] derivatives of *ortho*-carborane. Alternatively, hydrogen atoms bonded to the carbon atoms can also be replaced by halogen atoms. It should be noted that when substituted at a carbon atom, carborane acts as an electron-withdrawing group with respect to a substituent, while when substituted at boron atoms it plays the role of an electron-releasing group. The further the location of a substituent is from carbon atoms, the higher the electron-releasing ability is the carborane cage [35].

Halogen bonds are one of the strongest noncovalent intermolecular interactions, and are formed between the σ-hole of a halogen atom and nucleophile [36–39]. In the case of halogen bonds in which both atoms are halogens, the σ-hole is activated by electron acceptor substitution of a halogen while donor substituents are necessary to increase ability of lone pair donation of the second halogen atom. Therefore, in the case when halogen atoms are simultaneously introduced to the carborane carbon atom and the boron atom is antipodal to it, this makes the formation of intermolecular halogen bonds possible, where the halogen atom attached to the carbon atom plays the role of an acceptor, and the halogen atom bonded to boron acts as a donor. Thus, the *B,C*-dihalogen-substituted carboranes represent a unique class of small molecules, in the crystals of which the formation of intermolecular dihalogen bonds could be possible without the participation of the second component. In particular, one might expect a formation of the intermolecular dihalogen bonds for 1,12-dihalo-*ortho*-carboranes 1,12-X_2-1,2-$C_2B_{10}H_{10}$. However, the recent study of the crystal structure of 1,12-Br_2-1,2-$C_2B_{10}H_{10}$ showed that in this case, instead of the formation of the intermolecular C-Br··· Br-B dihalogen bonds, the formation of the C–H··· Br–B hydrogen and C-Br··· H-B halogen bonds occurs [28]. On the other hand, the σ-hole size, which is the determining factor in the formation of a halogen bond, depends on both the electronic effect of the substituent and the electronegativity of the halogen atom [40–42]. This prompted us to study intermolecular interactions in an analogous diiodine derivative 1,12-I_2-1,2-$C_2B_{10}H_{10}$ using single crystal X-ray diffraction and quantum chemical calculations.

2. Results and Discussion

Despite the fact that the syntheses of the *C*-iodo derivatives of *ortho*-carborane were first reported more than 50 years ago [43,44], they were on the periphery of mainstream carborane chemistry developments, and were not even well characterized [34,45]. In this way, they radically differ from the *B*-iodo derivatives of *ortho*-carborane, which have found active use in the synthesis of *B*-alkyl and aryl derivatives by means of Pd-catalyzed cross-coupling reactions [46–52]. Therefore, the synthesis of the *C*-iodo derivatives of *ortho*-carborane is not an easy task.

In this respect, the synthesis and characterization of the *C*-halogen derivatives of the carba-*closo*-dodecaborate anion $[1\text{-}X\text{-}1\text{-}CB_{11}H_{11}]^-$ (X = F, Cl, Br, I) are described much better [53]. Moreover, the preparation of its 1,12-diiodo derivative $[1,12\text{-}I_2\text{-}1\text{-}CB_{11}H_{10}]^-$, containing iodine atoms in opposite positions of the boron backbone, has recently been described [54]. However, in the case of anionic carboranes, it is rather difficult to find a cation that, on the one hand, will not form additional non-covalent bonds with the anion and, on the other hand, will be small enough not to hinder the formation of intermolecular dihalogen bonds between the anions. In addition, unlike the *C*-substituted *ortho*-carborane, the *C*-substituted carba-*closo*-dodecaborate anion has no or negligible electron-withdrawing effects [55].

An attempt to prepare 1,12-I_2-1,2-$C_2B_{10}H_{10}$ by the reaction of the lithium derivative of 9-iodo-*ortho*-carborane with iodine in 1,2-dimethoxyethane resulted in the expected formation of a mixture of 1,9-I_2-1,2-$C_2B_{10}H_{10}$ and 1,12-I_2-1,2-$C_2B_{10}H_{10}$ derivatives (1:1). However, in contrast to the similar dibromo derivatives 1,9-Br_2-1,2-$C_2B_{10}H_{10}$ and 1,12-Br_2-1,2-$C_2B_{10}H_{10}$ [56], we failed to separate this mixture. Nevertheless, we managed to obtain the desired 1,12-diiodo derivative as a by-product of the cross-coupling reaction of 9-iodo-*ortho*-carborane with phenylmagnesium bromide. Another by-product of this reaction was 1-iodo-*ortho*-carborane, which we also obtained by direct reaction of the lithium derivative of *ortho*-carborane with iodine. Notably, formation of similar products of iodine migration in the process of cross-coupling of *B*-iodo carboranes with Grignard reagents was noted earlier [57].

As mentioned in the Introduction, no Br··· Br halogen bond was observed in the crystal structure of 1,12-dibromo-*ortho*-carborane 1,12-Br_2-1,2-$C_2B_{10}H_{10}$ [28]. It should be noted that similarities and differences between bonding preferences of the bromine atom in comparison to iodine atom, on the one hand, and chlorine atom, on the other hand, was the subject of extensive studies [58–61]. Based on comparison of the crystal packing of 1-Ph-2-X-*ortho*-carboranes (X = F, Cl, Br, I), it was shown that both Br and I form Hal$\cdots\pi$ interactions, while neither Cl or F participate in such interactions [58]. Study of N-(2-halo-2,2-dinitroethyl)pyrrolidine- 2,5-diones (Hal = F, Cl, Br) [59] has revealed that both Cl and Br participate in halogen bonding, but bromine interacts with the carbonyl oxygen atom (the strongest donor site), while chlorine prefers to connect to much weaker donors, namely, oxygen atoms of the nitro group. Based on the above, it becomes unclear a priori which packing motif should be expected in the crystal of 1,12-diiodo-*ortho*-carborane.

Single crystals of 1,12-I_2-1,2-$C_2B_{10}H_{10}$ suitable for X-ray study were obtained in the form of thin plates by slow evaporation of chloroform solution. An asymmetric unit cell of 1,12-I_2-1,2-$C_2B_{10}H_{10}$ contains one molecule (Figure 1). The I1–C1 bond length (2.121(2) Å) is slightly longer than average X-ray value for I–C (aromatic) bonds (2.095 Å [62]) and is significantly shorter than the B12–I12 bond (2.179(2) Å).

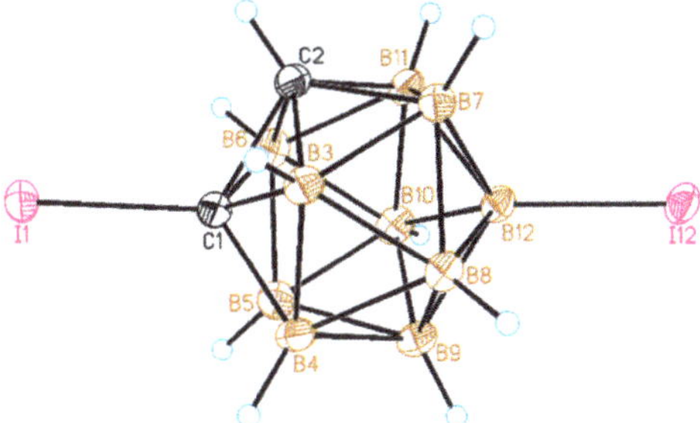

Figure 1. General view of 1,12-I_2-1,2-$C_2B_{10}H_{10}$. Thermal ellipsoids are given at 50% probability level.

The main packing motif of the crystal structure of 1,12-I_2-1,2-$C_2B_{10}H_{10}$ is represented by infinite chains along the *b* direction formed by the C–I$\cdots$I–B dihalogen bonds of II type [37,63] (the I(12)$\cdots$I(1′) distance is 3.5687(9) Å, the B(12)-I(12)$\cdots$I(1′) and I(12)$\cdots$I(1′)-C(1′) angles are 92.98(12) and 172.61(11)°, respectively) (Figure 2), which is very different from 1,12-Br_2-1,2-$C_2B_{10}H_{10}$ studied earlier.

In order to find out the reason of observed differences as well as peculiarities of the crystal packing of 1,12-I_2-1,2-$C_2B_{10}H_{10}$, we used energetic analysis of intermolecular contacts, that is frequently invoked for crystal packing study [64–66]. We calculated halogen bonded dimer for both compound 1,12-I_2-1,2-$C_2B_{10}H_{10}$ and similar dimer in which iodine atoms are replaced with bromines. The results are presented in Figure 3 and Table 1. The calculated dimer of 1,12-I_2-1,2-$C_2B_{10}H_{10}$ is characterized by the structure similar to that found experimentally. The I$\cdots$I distance is somewhat shorter, while C–I$\cdots$I and B–I$\cdots$I angles and B–H$\cdots$I distances are close to experimentally observed values. Topological analysis of calculated electron density for 1,12-I_2-1,2-$C_2B_{10}H_{10}$ dimer has revealed additional stabilization of the dimeric structure with the B–H$\cdots$I hydride–halogen bonds that was not evident from the consideration of bare X-ray data. From Table 1, it can be seen that energy of the I$\cdots$I contact is sizably higher than that of the B–H$\cdots$I contacts; therefore, the I$\cdots$I dihalogen bond can be considered as the structure-forming interaction in the crystal of 1,12-I_2-1,2-$C_2B_{10}H_{10}$. In contrary, optimized geometry of dimeric 1,12-dibromo-*ortho*-carborane appeared to be quite different. The C–Br$\cdots$Br angle significantly deviates from 180°. As a consequence, energy of the Br$\cdots$Br interactions is relatively small and becomes comparable to the B–H$\cdots$Br interactions which are also formed between two molecules in the dimer. It means that the Br$\cdots$Br interactions are no more structure-forming ones. These results are in qualitative agreement with a previous experiment [26]; according to which, no Br$\cdots$Br halogen bond is observed in the crystal of 1,12-Br_2-1,2-$C_2B_{10}H_{10}$.

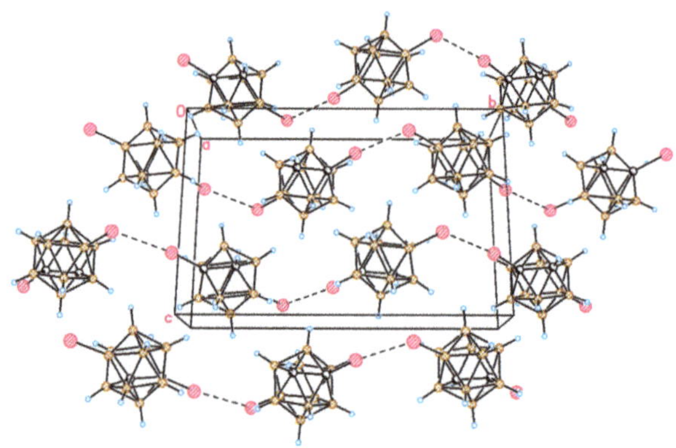

Figure 2. Crystal packing fragment of 1,12-I_2-1,2-$C_2B_{10}H_{10}$. Halogen bonded chains are formed along axis *b*.

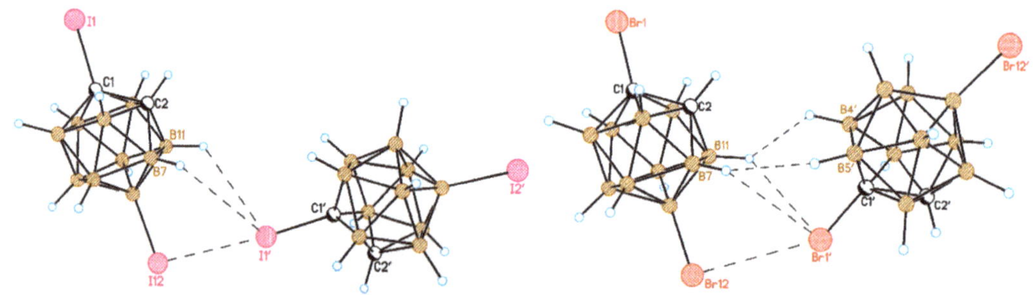

Figure 3. Noncovalent bonding in dimers of 1,12-I_2-1,2-$C_2B_{10}H_{10}$ (**left**) and 1,12-Br_2-1,2-$C_2B_{10}H_{10}$ (**right**).

Table 1. Characteristics of intermolecular noncovalent interactions for dimers of 1,12-I_2-1,2-$C_2B_{10}H_{10}$ and 1,12-Br_2-1,2-$C_2B_{10}H_{10}$.

	Distance in Å or Angle in Deg.			**Energy in kcal/mol**	
	1,12-I_2-1,2-$C_2B_{10}H_{10}$ (X-ray)	**1,12-I_2-1,2-$C_2B_{10}H_{10}$ (calc)**	**1,12-Br_2-1,2-$C_2B_{10}H_{10}$ (calc)**	**1,12-I_2-1,2-$C_2B_{10}H_{10}$ (calc)**	**1,12-Br_2-1,2-$C_2B_{10}H_{10}$ (calc)**
X12X1′	3.5687(9)	3.455	3.704	−2.9	−1.0
B12-X12· · ·X1′	92.98(12)	94.3	91.1		
X12· · ·X1′-C1′H7· · ·X1′	172.61(11)	175.9	147.6		
H11· · ·X1′	3.58(2)	3.51	3.25	−0.5	−0.7
H7· · ·H5′	3.58(2)	3.52	3.37	−0.5	−0.5
H11· · ·H4′	-	-	2.67	-	−0.5
X12X1′	-	-	2.61	-	−0.6

The above results have demonstrated computational ability for, at least, qualitative explanation and prediction of the main crystal packing motif for dihalogen derivatives of *ortho*-carborane. Based on that, we made an attempt to predict the possibility of halogen bond formation in 1,3-I_2-1,2-$C_2B_{10}H_{10}$ and 1,9-I_2-1,2-$C_2B_{10}H_{10}$. Those isomers were chosen because they can be experimentally obtained from the available 3- and 9-iodo-*ortho*-carboranes, while synthesis of other possible isomers is troublesome. In Figure 4 and Table 2, the results of calculation of dimers of the 1,3- and 1,9-isomers are presented.

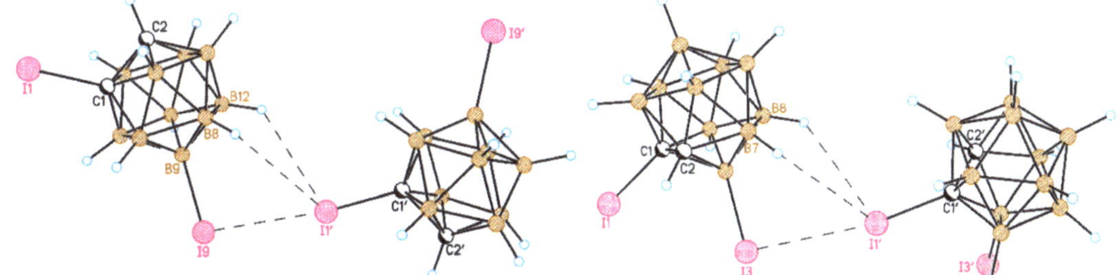

Figure 4. Noncovalent bonding in dimers of 1,9-I_2-1,2-$C_2B_{10}H_{10}$ (**left**) and 1,3-I_2-1,2-$C_2B_{10}H_{10}$ (**right**).

Table 2. Characteristics of intermolecular noncovalent interactions for halogen-bonded dimers of 1,3-I_2-1,2-$C_2B_{10}H_{10}$ and 1,9-I_2-1,2-$C_2B_{10}H_{10}$.

1,9-I_2-1,2-$C_2B_{10}H_{10}$			**1,3-I_2-1,2-$C_2B_{10}H_{10}$**		
	Distance or Angle	**Energy**		**Distance or Angle**	**Energy**
I9···I1′	3.461	−2.7	I3···I1′	3.54	−2.3
B9-I9···I1′	92.7		B3-I3···I1′	90.1	
I9···I1′-C1′	174.1		I3···I1′-C1′	170.7	
H12···I1′	3.47	−0.6	H8···I1′	3.44	−0.7
H8···I1′	3.49	−0.6	H10···I1′	3.42	−0.7

One can see that 1,9-I_2-1,2-$C_2B_{10}H_{10}$ demonstrates the same system of close contacts and nearly the same energetic properties of halogen-bonded dimer of 1,12-I_2-1,2-$C_2B_{10}H_{10}$. The energy of a halogen bond is only 0.2 kcal/mol less; B9-I9···I1′ and I9···I1′-C1′ only slightly deviate from 90 and 180°, respectively, while energies of B–H···I interactions are only 0.1 kcal/mol higher. It allows consideration of the I···I halogen bond as a predominant interaction in the potential crystal structure of 1,9-I_2-1,2-$C_2B_{10}H_{10}$.

When looking at halogen-bonded dimers built up of 1,3-I_2-1,2-$C_2B_{10}H_{10}$, one can observe a clear trend of weakening of the I···I halogen bonds and simultaneous strengthening of the B–H···I interactions and increases in their roles in stabilizing dimeric structures upon approaching the iodine substituent from its position at B12 to B3. During movement of the iodine atom from B12 to B3, quantitative changes due to the weakening of the I···I halogen bonds can be transformed to qualitative changes, which can result in the disappearance of the I···I halogen bonds from the crystal structure of 1,3-I_2-1,2-$C_2B_{10}H_{10}$.

In conclusion, 1,12-diiodo-*ortho*-carborane was obtained and its crystal structure was determined by X-ray diffraction, which revealed the existence of the I···I halogen bond in its crystal structure, in contrast to 1,12-dibromo-*ortho*-carborane. Based on quantum chemical calculation, we have determined preferences of the type of noncovalent interactions in 1,12-diiodo- and 1,12-dibromo-*ortho*-carboranes which appeared to be in agreement with experimental findings. Based on our results, we can predict the formation of the I···I halogen bonds in 1,9-diiodo-*ortho*-carborane, while our results cannot provide solid support for the formation of such bonds in the 1,3-isomer. This question is still open and can be answered experimentally. Synthesis and crystal growth of 1,9- and 1,3-diiodo-*ortho*-carboranes is in progress in our group.

3. Materials and Methods

3.1. General

Compounds 9-iodo-*ortho*-carborane and bis(triphenylphosphine)palladium(II) dichloride were prepared according to the literature procedures [67,68]. Solvents 1,2-dimethoxyethane and diethyl ether were dried using standard procedures [69]. Phenyl iodide was distilled at boiling point. All other chemical reagents were purchased from Sigma Aldrich, Acros

Organics and ABCR and used without purification. All reactions were carried out in an argon atmosphere. The reaction progress was monitored by thin-layer chromatography (Merck F254 silica gel on aluminum plates) and visualized using 0.5% $PdCl_2$ in 1% HCl in aq. MeOH (1:10). Acros Organics silica gel (0.060–0.200 mm) was used for column chromatography. The NMR spectra at 400.1 MHz (^{1}H), 128.4 MHz (^{11}B) and 100.0 MHz (^{13}C) were recorded with a Varian Inova 400 spectrometer. The residual signal of the NMR solvent relative to Me_4Si was taken as an internal reference for ^{1}H and ^{13}C NMR spectra; ^{11}B NMR spectra were referenced using $BF_3{\cdot}Et_2O$ as an external standard.

3.2. Cross-Coupling of 9-Iodo-Ortho-Carborane with PhMgBr

Phenyl iodide (0.70 mL, 1275 mg, 6.25 mmol) was added to a mixture of magnesium turnings (228 mg, 9.38 mmol) in fresh distilled diethyl ether (25 mL). The resulting mixture was heated under reflux for 1 h. Then, 9-iodo-*ortho*-carborane (675 mg, 2.50 mmol) in fresh distilled diethyl ether (25 mL) was added, and the reaction was stirred at room temperature for another 1 h. Then, copper(I) iodide (25 mg, 0.13 mmol, catalytic amount) with $[(Ph_3P)_2PdCl_2]$ (83 mg, 0.13 mmol, catalytic amount) were added. The reaction was heated under reflux for 16 h and 6% HCl in water (50 mL) was added. The organic layer was separated; the water layer was washed with diethyl ether (3 × 50 mL). The organic phases were combined, dried over Na_2SO_4, and concentrated under reduced pressure. The crude product was purified by column chromatography on silica using a mixture of chloroform and petroleum ether (1:3, v/v) to give, along with the expected 9-phenyl-*ortho*-carborane, pale-yellow solids of 1-iodo-*ortho*-carborane (15 mg, yield 2%) and 1,12-diiodo-*ortho*- carborane (20 mg, yield 2%) as side products.

Compound 1-I-1,2-$C_2B_{10}H_{11}$: ^{1}H NMR ($CDCl_3$, ppm): δ 3.78 (1H, br s, CH_{carb}), 3.7–0.7 (10H, br m, *BH*). ^{11}B NMR ($CDCl_3$, ppm): δ −0.7 (1B, d, J = 151 Hz), −4.0 (1B, d, J = 154 Hz), −7.8 (4B, d, J = 125 Hz), −9.0 (2B, d, J = 111 Hz), −11.7 (1B, d, J = 167 Hz).

Compound 1,12-I_2-1,2-$C_2B_{10}H_{10}$: ^{1}H NMR ($CDCl_3$, ppm): δ 3.86 (1H, br s, CH_{carb}), 4.1–0.6 (9H, br m, *BH*). ^{11}B NMR ($CDCl_3$, ppm): δ 0.9 (1B, d, J = 156 Hz), –5.8 (2B, d, J = 160 Hz), −7.8 (2B, d, J = 173 Hz), −8.7 (2B, d, J = 183 Hz), −10.7 (2B, d, J = 168 Hz), −16.7 (1B, s).

3.3. General Synthetic Procedure of C-Iodination of Ortho-Carborane and Its B-I Derivatives

The 2.25 M BuLi in hexanes was added to a mixture of carborane in fresh distilled 1,2-dimethoxyethane (10 mL). The mixture was stirred for 1 h at room temperature and I_2 was added by one portion. The reaction was stirred at room temperature overnight and $Na_2S_2O_3{\cdot}5H_2O$ (1000 g, 4.03 mmol) in water (10 mL) and diethyl ether (15 mL) were added. The organic layer was separated; the water layer was washed with diethyl ether (25 mL). The organic phases were combined, dried over Na_2SO_4, and concentrated under reduced pressure. The crude product was purified by column chromatography on silica using diethyl ether as the eluent to give the corresponding C–I derivative.

Compound 1,2-I_2-1,2-$C_2B_{10}H_{10}$: 2.25 M BuLi in hexanes (1.00 mL, 2.25 mmol), *ortho*-carborane (144 mg, 1.00 mmol) and I_2 (635 mg, 2.50 mmol) were used; a yellow crystalline solid was obtained (381 mg, yield 96%). ^{1}H NMR ($CDCl_3$, ppm): δ 3.9–0.8 (10H, br m, *BH*). ^{11}B NMR ($CDCl_3$, ppm): δ −2.5 (2B, d, J = 154 Hz), −4.5 (2B, d, J = 183 Hz), −6.8 (6B, d, J = 183 Hz).

Compounds 1,9- and 1,12-I_2-1,2-$C_2B_{10}H_{10}$: 2.25 M BuLi in hexanes (0.49 mL, 1.10 mmol), 9-iodo-*ortho*-carborane (135 mg, 0.50 mmol) and I_2 (305 mg, 1.20 mmol) were used; a pale-grey crystalline solid was obtained (80 mg, yield 20%). ^{1}H NMR ($CDCl_3$, ppm): δ 4.07 (1H, br s, CH_{carb}, 1,9-isomer), 3.87 (1H, br s, CH_{carb}, 1,12-isomer), 3.9–0.6 (20H, br m, *BH*, 1,9 + 1,12-isomers).

3.4. Synthesis of 1-Iodo-Ortho-Carborane

The 2.25 M BuLi in hexanes (0.40 mL, 0.90 mmol) was added to a mixture of *ortho*-carborane (144 mg, 1.00 mmol) in fresh distilled 1,2-dimethoxyethane (10 mL). The mixture was stirred for 1 h at room temperature, and I_2 (381 mg, 1.50 mmol) was added by one portion. The reaction was stirred at room temperature overnight and $Na_2S_2O_3{\cdot}5H_2O$ (1000 g, 4.03 mmol) in water (10 mL) and diethyl ether (15 mL) were added. The organic layer was separated; the water layer was washed with diethyl ether (25 mL). The organic phases were combined, dried over Na_2SO_4, and concentrated under reduced pressure. The crude product was purified by column chromatography on silica using petroleum ether as an eluent to give a pale-grey crystalline solid of 1-I-1,2-$C_2B_{10}H_{11}$ (160 mg, yield 59%).

3.5. X-ray Diffraction Study

Single crystal X-ray diffraction experiments were carried out using a SMART APEX2 CCD diffractometer (λ(Mo-Kα) = 0.71073 Å, graphite monochromator, ω-scans) at 120 K. Collected data were processed by the SAINT and SADABS programs incorporated into the APEX2 program package [70]. The structures were solved by the direct methods and refined by the full-matrix least-squares procedure against F^2 in anisotropic approximation. The refinement was carried out with the SHELXTL program [71]. The CCDC numbers (2070233 for 1,12-I_2-$C_2B_{10}H_{10}$ and 2074102 for 1-I-$C_2B_{10}H_{11}$) contain the supplementary crystallographic data for this paper. These data can be found in the Supplementary Materials or obtained free of charge via www.ccdc.cam.ac.uk/data_request/cif, accessed on 15 March 2021.

Crystallographic data for 1,12-I_2-1,2-$C_2B_{10}H_{10}$: $C_2H_{10}B_{10}I_2$ are monoclinic, space group $P2_1/c$: a = 7.1919(8)Å, b = 15.8202(17)Å, c = 11.1509(12)Å, β = 108.809(2)°, V = 1201.0(2) Å^3, Z = 4, M = 396.00, d_{cryst} = 2.190 g·cm^{-3}. $wR2$ = 0.0365 calculated on F^2_{hkl} for all 3557 independent reflections with $2\theta < 60.4°$, (GOF = 1.067, R = 0.0161 calculated on F_{hkl} for 3314 reflections with $I > 2\sigma(I)$).

Crystallographic data for 1-I-1,2-$C_2B_{10}H_{11}$: $C_2H_{11}B_{10}I$ are orthorhombic, space group $Pnma$: a = 13.8323(9)Å, b = 8.9644(6)Å, c = 8.4539(5)Å, V = 1048.27(12) Å^3, Z = 4, M = 270.11, d_{cryst} = 1.711 g·cm^{-3}. $wR2$ = 0.0747 calculated on F^2_{hkl} for all 1344 independent reflections with $2\theta < 56.1°$, (GOF = 1.143, R = 0.0327 calculated on F_{hkl} for 1203 reflections with $I > 2\sigma(I)$).

3.6. Quantum Chemical Calculations

All quantum chemical calculations were carried out with the Gaussian09 program [72]. The PBE0 functional with the triple zeta basis set was found to be reliable for the calculation of noncovalent intra- and intermolecular interactions [73–75] and was adopted throughout this study. Initial geometries for the optimization of all dimers considered in this study were based on the X-ray structure of a dihalogen-bonded dimer of 1,12-I_2-$C_2B_{10}H_{10}$ (symmetry code is 1 − x, −0.5 + y, 0.5 − z). All dimeric associates were fully optimized and converged to the energy minima. Theoretical electron density was treated within the AIM approach [76] using the AIMAll program package [77]. For energy (E) estimation, we used the $E = 1/2V(r)$ formula [78,79], in which $V(r)$ is the potential energy density at the bond critical point between interacting atoms. It has frequently been shown that this approach to describe noncovalent interactions demonstrates realistic energetic characteristics [80–82].

Supplementary Materials: The following are available online at https://www.mdpi.com/article/10.3390/cryst11040396/s1, Figure S1: Asymmetric part of 1-I-1,2-$C_2B_{10}H_{11}$ molecule showing numbering scheme and the disorder of the C2/B4 atoms; Figure S2: General view of 1-I-1,2-$C_2B_{10}H_{11}$; Figure S3: Halogen bonded dimer of 1-I-1,2-$C_2B_{10}H_{11}$, and complete crystallographic data (cif-files) for compounds 1-I-1,2-$C_2B_{10}H_{11}$ and 1,12-I_2-1,2-$C_2B_{10}H_{10}$.

Author Contributions: Synthesis and NMR spectroscopy study, S.A.A.; quantum-chemical calculations, A.A.A.; X-ray diffraction experiment and final manuscript writing, K.Y.S.; general manuscript concept and final manuscript writing, I.B.S.; technical editing, V.I.B. All authors have read and agreed to the published version of the manuscript.

Funding: This research was supported by the Russian Science Foundation—synthesis by Grant No. 19-73-00353 and crystal packing analysis and quantum-chemical calculations by Grant No. 19-13-00238.

Institutional Review Board Statement: Not applicable.

Informed Consent Statement: Not applicable.

Data Availability Statement: The supporting data are available on request from the authors.

Acknowledgments: The NMR spectroscopy and X-ray diffraction data were obtained by using equipment from the Center for Molecular Structure Studies at A.N. Nesmeyanov Institute of Organoelement Compounds, operating with support from the Ministry of Science and Higher Education of the Russian Federation.

Conflicts of Interest: The authors declare no conflict of interest. The funders had no role in the design of the study; in the collection, analyses, or interpretation of data; in the writing of the manuscript, or in the decision to publish the results.

References

1. Grimes, R.N. *Carboranes*, 3rd ed.; Academic Press: London, UK, 2016; 1042p. [CrossRef]
2. Kaszynski, P.; Douglass, A.G. Organic derivatives of closo-boranes: A new class of liquid crystal materials. *J. Organomet. Chem.* **1999**, *581*, 28–38. [CrossRef]
3. Pecyna, J.; Pociecha, D.; Kaszynski, P. Zwitterionic pyridinium derivatives of [closo-1- CB_9H_{10}]- and [closo-1-$CB_{11}H_{12}$]- as high $\Delta\varepsilon$ additives to a nematic host. *J. Mater. Chem. C* **2014**, *2*, 1585–1591. [CrossRef]
4. Pecyna, J.; Kaszyński, P.; Ringstrand, B.; Pociecha, D.; Pakhomov, S.; Douglass, A.G.; Young, V.G. Synthesis and characterization of quinuclidinium derivatives of the [closo-1-$CB_{11}H_{12}$]-anion as potential polar components of liquid crystal materials. *Inorg. Chem.* **2016**, *55*, 40167–44025. [CrossRef]
5. Pecyna, J.; Jankowiak, A.; Pociecha, D.; Kaszyński, P. o-Carborane derivatives for probing molecular polarity effects on liquid crystal phase stability and dielectric behavior. *J. Mater. Chem. C* **2015**, *3*, 11412–11422. [CrossRef]
6. Allis, D.G.; Spencer, J.T. Polyhedral-based nonlinear optical materials. 2. Theoretical investigation of some new high non-linear optical response compounds involving polyhedral bridges with charged aromatic donors and acceptors. *Inorg. Chem.* **2001**, *40*, 3373–3380. [CrossRef]
7. Wang, H.-Q.; Wang, L.; Li, R.-R.; Ye, J.-T.; Chen, Z.-Z.; Chen, H.; Qiu, Y.-Q.; Xie, H.-M. Second-order nonlinear optical properties of carboranylated square-planar Pt(II) zwitterionic complexes: One-/two-dimensional difference and substituent effect. *J. Phys. Chem. A* **2016**, *120*, 9330–9340. [CrossRef] [PubMed]
8. Jiang, P.; Wang, Z.; Moxey, G.J.; Morshedi, M.; Barlow, A.; Wang, G.; Quintana, C.; Zhang, C.; Cifuentes, M.P.; Humphrey, M.G. Syntheses and quadratic nonlinear optical properties of 2,7-fluorenylene- and 1,4-phenylene-functionalized o-carboranes. *Dalton Trans.* **2019**, *48*, 12549–12559. [CrossRef] [PubMed]
9. Wang, H.-Q.; Ye, J.-T.; Zhang, Y.; Zhao, Y.-Y.; Qiu, Y.-Q. A thorough understanding of the nonlinear optical properties of BODIPY/carborane/diketopyrrolopyrrole hybrid chromophores: Module contribution, linear combination, one-/two-dimensional difference and carborane's arrangement. *J. Mater. Chem. C* **2019**, *7*, 7531–7547. [CrossRef]
10. Wedge, T.J.; Hawthorne, M. Multidentate carborane-containing Lewis acids and their chemistry: Mercuracarborands. *Coord. Chem. Rev.* **2003**, *240*, 111–128. [CrossRef]
11. Scholz, M.; Hey-Hawkins, E. Carbaboranes as Pharmacophores: Properties, Synthesis, and Application Strategies. *Chem. Rev.* **2011**, *111*, 7035–7062. [CrossRef] [PubMed]
12. Endo, Y. Carboranes as hydrophobic pharmacophores: Applications for design of nuclear receptor ligands. In *Boron-Based Compounds: Potential and Emerging Applications in Medicine*; Hey-Hawkins, E., Viñas Teixidor, C., Eds.; John Wiley & Sons Ltd.: Oxford, UK, 2018; pp. 3–19. [CrossRef]
13. Yang, X.; Jiang, W.; Knobler, C.B.; Hawthorne, M.F. Rigid-rod molecules: Carborods. Synthesis of tetrameric p-carboranes and the crystal structure of bis(tri-n-butylsilyl)tetra-p-carborane. *J. Am. Chem. Soc.* **1992**, *114*, 9719–9721. [CrossRef]
14. Schöberl, U.; Magnera, T.F.; Harrison, R.M.; Fleischer, F.; Pflug, J.L.; Schwab, P.F.H.; Meng, X.; Lipiak, D.; Noll, B.C.; Allured, V.S.; et al. Toward a Hexagonal Grid Polymer: Synthesis, Coupling, and Chemically Reversible Surface-Pinning of the Star Connectors, 1,3,5-$C_6H_3(CB_{10}H_{10}CX)_3$. *J. Am. Chem. Soc.* **1997**, *119*, 3907–3917. [CrossRef]
15. Fox, M.A.; Cameron, A.M.; Low, P.J.; Paterson, M.A.J.; Batsanov, A.S.; Goeta, A.E.; Rankin, D.W.H.; Robertson, H.E.; Schirlin, J.T. Synthetic and structural studies on C-ethynyl- and C-bromo-carboranes. *Dalton Trans.* **2006**, 3544–3560. [CrossRef] [PubMed]
16. Safronov, A.V.; Sevryugina, Y.V.; Pichaandi, K.R.; Jalisatgi, S.S.; Hawthorne, M.F. Synthesis of closo- and nido-biscarboranes with rigid unsaturated linkers as precursors to linear metallacarborane-based molecular rods. *Dalton Trans.* **2014**, *43*, 4969–4977. [CrossRef]
17. Himmelspach, A.; Warneke, J.; Schäfer, M.; Hailmann, M.; Finze, M. Salts of the dianions [Hg(12-X-closo-1-$CB_{11}H_{10})_2]_2$- (X = I, C≡CH, C≡CFc, C≡CSiiPr$_3$): Synthesis and spectroscopic and structural characterization. *Organometallics* **2015**, *34*, 462–469. [CrossRef]
18. Zhang, K.; Shen, Y.; Liu, J.; Spingler, B.; Duttwyler, S. Crystal structure of a carborane endo/exo-dianion and its use in the synthesis of ditopic ligands for supramolecular frameworks. *Chem. Commun.* **2017**, *54*, 1698–1701. [CrossRef] [PubMed]

19. Farha, O.K.; Spokoyny, A.M.; Mulfort, K.L.; Hawthorne, M.F.; Mirkin, C.A.; Hupp, J.T. Synthesis and Hydrogen Sorption Properties of Carborane Based Metal–Organic Framework Materials. *J. Am. Chem. Soc.* **2007**, *129*, 12680–12681. [CrossRef]
20. Bae, Y.-S.; Farha, O.K.; Spokoyny, A.M.; Mirkin, C.A.; Hupp, J.T.; Snurr, R.Q. Carborane-based metal–organic frameworks as highly selective sorbents for CO_2 over methane. *Chem. Commun.* **2008**, 4135–4137. [CrossRef]
21. Bae, Y.-S.; Spokoyny, A.M.; Farha, O.K.; Snurr, R.Q.; Hupp, J.T.; Mirkin, C.A. Separation of gas mixtures using Co(II) car-borane-based porous coordination polymers. *Chem. Commun.* **2010**, *46*, 3478–3480. [CrossRef]
22. Kennedy, R.D.; Krungleviciute, V.; Clingerman, D.J.; Mondloch, J.E.; Peng, Y.; Wilmer, C.E.; Sarjeant, A.A.; Snurr, R.Q.; Hupp, J.T.; Yildirim, T.; et al. Carborane-based metal-organic framework with high methane and hydrogen storage capacities. *Chem. Mater.* **2013**, *25*, 3539–3543. [CrossRef]
23. Andrews, P.; Hardie, M.J.; Raston, C.L. Supramolecular assemblies of globular main group cage species. *Coord. Chem. Rev.* **1999**, *189*, 169–198. [CrossRef]
24. Hardie, M.J.; Raston, C.L. Crystalline hydrogen bonded complexes of o-carborane. *CrystEngComm* **2001**, *3*, 162–164. [CrossRef]
25. Lo, R.; Fanfrlík, J.; Lepšík, M.; Hobza, P. The properties of substituted 3D-aromatic neutral carboranes: The potential for σ-hole bonding. *Phys. Chem. Chem. Phys.* **2015**, *17*, 20814–20821. [CrossRef]
26. Alkorta, I.; Elguero, J.; Oliva-Enrich, J.M. Hydrogen vs. Halogen Bonds in 1-Halo-Closo-Carboranes. *Materials* **2020**, *13*, 2163. [CrossRef] [PubMed]
27. Glukhov, I.V.; Lyssenko, K.A.; Antipin, M.Y. Crystal packing of 8,9,10,12-tetrafluoro-o-carborane: H. F versus H. H contacts. *Struct. Chem.* **2007**, *18*, 465–469. [CrossRef]
28. Fanfrlík, J.; Holub, J.; Růžičková, Z.; Řezáč, J.; Lane, P.D.; Wann, D.A.; Hnyk, D.; Růžička, A.; Hobza, P. Competition between Halogen, Hydrogen and Dihydrogen Bonding in Brominated Carboranes. *ChemPhysChem* **2016**, *17*, 3373–3376. [CrossRef]
29. Batsanov, A.S.; Fox, M.A.; Howard, J.A.K.; Hughes, A.K.; Johnson, A.L.; Martindale, S.J. 9,12-diiodo-1,2-dicarba-closo-dodecaborane(12). *Acta Crystallogr. Sect. C Cryst. Struct. Commun.* **2003**, *59*, o74–o76. [CrossRef] [PubMed]
30. Barberà, G.; Viñas, C.; Teixidor, F.; Rosair, G.M.; Welch, A.J. Self-assembly of carborane molecules via C-H . . . I hydrogen bonding: The molecular and crystal structures of 3-I-1,2-closo-C2B10H11. *J. Chem. Soc. Dalton Trans.* **2002**, *19*, 3647–3648. [CrossRef]
31. Vaca, A.; Teixidor, F.; Kivekäs, R.; Sillanpää, R.; Viñas, C. A solvent-free regioselective iodination route of ortho-carboranes. *Dalton Trans.* **2006**, *41*, 4884–4885. [CrossRef]
32. Ramachandran, B.M.; Knobler, C.B.; Hawthorne, M.F. Synthesis and structural characterization of symmetrical clo-so-4,7-I2-1,2-$C_2B_{10}H_{10}$ and [$(CH_3)_3$NH][nido-2,4-I2-7,8-$C_2B_9H_{10}$]. *Inorg. Chem.* **2006**, *45*, 336–340. [CrossRef]
33. Barberà, G.; Vaca, A.; Teixidor, F.; Sillanpää, R.; Kivekäs, R.; Viñas, C. Designed synthesis of new ortho-carborane derivatives: From mono- to polysubstituted frameworks. *Inorg. Chem.* **2008**, *47*, 7309–7316. [CrossRef]
34. Puga, A.V.; Teixidor, F.; Sillanpää, R.; Kivekäs, R.; Viñas, C. Iodinated ortho-carboranes as versatile building blocks to design intermolecular interactions in crystal lattices. *Chem. Eur. J.* **2009**, *15*, 9764–9772. [CrossRef]
35. Bregadze, V.I. Dicarba-closo-dodecaboranes $C_2B_{10}H_{12}$ and their derivatives. *Chem. Rev.* **1992**, *92*, 209–223. [CrossRef]
36. Clark, T.; Hennemann, M.; Murray, J.S.; Politzer, P. Halogen bonding: The σ-hole. *J. Mol. Model.* **2007**, *13*, 291–296. [CrossRef]
37. Cavallo, G.; Metrangolo, P.; Milani, R.; Pilati, T.; Priimagi, A.; Resnati, G.; Terraneo, G. The Halogen Bond. *Chem. Rev.* **2016**, *116*, 2478–2601. [CrossRef] [PubMed]
38. Kolář, M.H.; Hobza, P. Computer Modeling of Halogen Bonds and Other σ-Hole Interactions. *Chem. Rev.* **2016**, *116*, 5155–5187. [CrossRef] [PubMed]
39. Gilday, L.C.; Robinson, S.W.; Barendt, T.A.; Langton, M.J.; Mullaney, B.R.; Beer, P.D. Halogen Bonding in Supramolecular Chemistry. *Chem. Rev.* **2015**, *115*, 7118–7195. [CrossRef]
40. Kolář, M.; Hostaš, J.; Hobza, P. The strength and directionality of a halogen bond are co-determined by the magnitude and size of the σ-hole. *Phys. Chem. Chem. Phys.* **2014**, *16*, 9987–9996. [CrossRef] [PubMed]
41. Ivanov, D.M.; Kinzhalov, M.A.; Novikov, A.S.; Ananyev, I.V.; Romanova, A.A.; Boyarskiy, V.P.; Haukka, M.; Kukushkin, V.Y. H2C(X)–X···X– (X = Cl, Br) Halogen Bonding of Dihalomethanes. *Cryst. Growth Des.* **2017**, *17*, 1353–1362. [CrossRef]
42. Suponitsky, K.Y.; Burakov, N.; Kanibolotsky, A.L.; Mikhailov, V.A. Multiple Noncovalent Bonding in Halogen Complexes with Oxygen Organics. I. Tertiary Amides. *J. Phys. Chem. A* **2016**, *120*, 4179–4190. [CrossRef]
43. Zakharkin, L.I.; Zhigareva, G.G.; Kazantsev, A.V. Some reactions of barene Gringard reagents. *Zh. Obshch. Khim.* **1968**, *38*, 89–92.
44. Zakharkin, L.I.; Podvisotskaya, L.S. Cleavage of 1,2-dihalobarenes by alcohols to C,C?-dihalodicarbaundecaboranes (13). *Russ. Chem. Bull.* **1966**, *15*, 742. [CrossRef]
45. Tupchauskas, A.P.; Stanko, V.I.; Ustynyuk, Y.A.; Khrapov, V.V. 1H-{11B} heteronuclear double resonance spectra of ortho-, meta-, and para-carboranes and some of their organotin derivatives. *J. Struct. Chem.* **1973**, *13*, 772–776. [CrossRef]
46. Zakharkin, L.; Kovredov, A.; Ol'Shevskaya, V.; Shaugumbekova, Z. Synthesis of B-organo-substituted 1,2-, 1,7-, and 1,12-dicarbaclosododecarboranes(12). *J. Organomet. Chem.* **1982**, *226*, 217–222. [CrossRef]
47. Zakharkin, L.I.; Ol'Shevskaya, V.A.; Nesmeyanov'S, A.N. Synthesis of 9-Organyl-1,2 and 1,7-Dicarba-closo-dodecaboranss(12) via the Cross-Coupling Reactions between Organozinc Compounds and 9-Iodo-1,2- or 1,7-Dicarba-closo-dodecaboranes. *Synth. React. Inorg. Met. Chem.* **1991**, *21*, 1041–1046. [CrossRef]
48. Zheng, Z.; Jiang, W.; Zinn, A.A.; Knobler, C.B.; Hawthorne, M.F. Facile Electrophilic Iodination of Icosahedral Carboranes. Synthesis of Carborane Derivatives with Boron-Carbon Bonds via the Palladium-Catalyzed Reaction of Diiodocarboranes with Grignard Reagents. *Inorg. Chem.* **1995**, *34*, 2095–2100. [CrossRef]

49. Viñas, C.; Barbera, G.; Oliva, J.M.; Teixidor, F.; Welch, A.J.; Rosair, G.M. Are halocarboranes suitable for substitution reactions? The case for 3-I-1,2-closo-$C_2B_{10}H_{11}$: Molecular orbital calculations, aryldehalogenation reactions, ^{11}B NMR interpretation of closo-carboranes, and molecular structures of 1-Ph-3-Br-1,2-closo-$C_2B_{10}H_{10}$ and 3-Ph-1,2-closo-$C_2B_{10}H_{11}$. *Inorg. Chem.* **2001**, *40*, 6555–6562. [CrossRef] [PubMed]
50. Endo, Y.; Aizawa, K.; Ohta, K. Synthesis of 3-Aryl-1,2-dicarba-closo-dodecaboranes by Suzuki-Miyaura Coupling Reaction. *Heterocycles* **2010**, *80*, 369–377. [CrossRef]
51. Anderson, K.P.; Mills, H.A.; Mao, C.; Kirlikovali, K.O.; Axtell, J.C.; Rheingold, A.L.; Spokoyny, A.M. Improved synthesis of icosahedral carboranes containing exopolyhedral B C and C C bonds. *Tetrahedron* **2019**, *75*, 187–191. [CrossRef]
52. Anufriev, S.A.; Shmal'ko, A.V.; Suponitsky, K.Y.; Sivaev, I.B. One-pot synthesis of B-aryl carboranes with sensitive functional groups using sequential cobalt- and palladium-catalyzed reactions. *Catalysts* **2020**, *10*, 1348. [CrossRef]
53. Janoušek, Z.; Hilton, C.L.; Schreiber, P.J.; Michl, J. C-Halogenation of the closo-$[CB_{11}H_{12}]^-$ Anion. *Collect. Czechoslov. Chem. Commun.* **2002**, *67*, 1025–1034. [CrossRef]
54. Šembera, F.; Plutnar, J.; Higelin, A.; Janoušek, Z.; Císařova, I.; Michl, J. Metal complexes with very large dipole moments: The anionic carborane nitriles 12-NC-$CB_{11}X_{11}^-$ (X = H, F, CH_3) as ligands on Pt(II) and Pd(II). *Inorg. Chem.* **2016**, *55*, 3797–3806. [CrossRef]
55. Estrada, J.; Lugo, C.A.; McArthur, S.G.; Lavallo, V. Inductive effects of 10 and 12-vertex closo-carborane anions: Cluster size and charge make a difference. *Chem. Commun.* **2016**, *52*, 1824–1826. [CrossRef] [PubMed]
56. Plešek, J.; Hanslík, T. Chemistry of boranes. XXIX. The synthesis of isomeric 1,9- and 1,12-dibromo- 1,2-dicarba-closo-dodecaboranes. *Collect. Czechoslov. Chem. Commun.* **1973**, *38*, 335–337. [CrossRef]
57. Anufriev, S.A.; Sivaev, I.B.; Bregadze, V.I. Synthesis of 9,9′,12,12′-substituted cobalt bis(dicarbollide) derivatives. *Russ. Chem. Bull.* **2015**, *64*, 712–717. [CrossRef]
58. Havránek, M.; Samsonov, M.A.; Holub, J.; Ružickova, Z.; Drož, L.; Ružicka, A.; Fanfrlík, J.; Hnyk, D. The influence of halogenated hypercarbon on crystal packing in the series of 1-Ph-2-X-1,2-dicarba-closo-dodecaboranes (X = F, Cl, Br, I). *Molecules* **2020**, *25*, 1200. [CrossRef]
59. Dmitrienko, A.O.; Karnoukhova, V.A.; Potemkin, A.A.; Struchkova, M.I.; Kryazhevskikh, I.A.; Suponitsky, K.Y. The influence of halogen type on structural features of compounds containing α-halo-α,α-dinitroethyl moieties. *Chem. Heterocycl. Comp.* **2017**, *53*, 532–539. [CrossRef]
60. Wolff, M.; Okrut, A.; Feldmann, C. $[(Ph)_3PBr][Br_3]$, $[(Bz)(Ph)_3P]_2[Br_8]$, $[(n\text{-}Bu)_3MeN]_2[Br_{20}]$, $[C_4MPyr]_2[Br_{20}]$, and $[(Ph)_3PCl]_2[Cl_2I_{14}]$: Extending the Horizon of Polyhalides via Synthesis in Ionic Liquids. *Inorg. Chem.* **2011**, *50*, 11683–11694. [CrossRef]
61. Sonnenberg, K.; Mann, L.; Redeker, F.A.; Schmidt, B.; Riedel, S. Polyhalogen and Polyinterhalogen Anions from Fluorine to Iodine. *Angew. Chem. Int. Ed.* **2020**, *59*, 5464–5493. [CrossRef]
62. Allen, F.H.; Kennard, O.; Watson, D.G.; Brammer, L.; Orpen, A.G.; Taylor, R. Tables of bond lengths determined by X-ray and neutron diffraction. Part 1. Bond lengths in organic compounds. *J. Chem. Soc. Perkin Trans.* **1987**, *2*, S1–S19. [CrossRef]
63. Varadwaj, P.R.; Varadwaj, A.; Marques, H.M. Halogen bonding: A halogen-centered noncovalent interaction yet to be understood. *Inorganics* **2019**, *7*, 40. [CrossRef]
64. Suponitsky, K.Y.; Tsirelson, V.G.; Feil, D. Electron-density-based calculations of intermolecular energy: Case of urea. *Acta Crystallogr. Sect. A Found. Crystallogr.* **1999**, *55*, 821–827. [CrossRef] [PubMed]
65. Suponitsky, K.Y.; Smol'Yakov, A.F.; Ananyev, I.V.; Khakhalev, A.V.; Gidaspov, A.A.; Sheremetev, A.B. 3,4-Dinitrofurazan: Structural Nonequivalence of ortho -Nitro Groups as a Key Feature of the Crystal Structure and Density. *ChemistrySelect* **2020**, *5*, 14543–14548. [CrossRef]
66. Dalinger, I.L.; Suponitsky, K.Y.; Pivkina, A.N.; Sheremetev, A.B. Novel melt-castable energetic pyrazole: A pyrazol-yl-furazan framework bearing five nitro groups. *Prop. Explos. Pyrotech.* **2016**, *41*, 789–792. [CrossRef]
67. Andrews, J.S.; Zayas, J.; Jones, M. 9-Iodo-o-carborane. *Inorg. Chem.* **1985**, *24*, 3715–3716. [CrossRef]
68. Itatani, H.; Bailar, J.C. Homogenous catalysis in the reactions of olefinic substances. V. Hydrogenation of soybean oil methyl ester with triphenylphosphine and triphenylarsine palladium catalysts. *J. Am. Oil Chem. Soc.* **1967**, *44*, 147–151. [CrossRef]
69. Armarego, W.L.F.; Chai, C.L.L. *Purification of Laboratory Chemicals*, 6th ed.; Butterworth-Heinemann: Burlington, NJ, USA, 2009. [CrossRef]
70. Bruker AXS. *APEX2 and SAINT*; Bruker AXS Inc.: Madison, WI, USA, 2014.
71. Sheldrick, G.M. Crystal structure refinement with SHELXL. *Acta Cryst.* **2015**, *71*, 3–8. [CrossRef]
72. Frisch, M.J.; Trucks, G.W.; Schlegel, H.B.; Scuseria, G.E.; Robb, M.A.; Cheeseman, J.R.; Montgomery, J.A.; Kudin, K.N., Jr.; Burant, J.C.; Millam, J.M.; et al. *Gaussian 03, Revision E.01*; Gaussian, Inc.: Wallingford, UK, 2004.
73. Anufriev, S.A.; Sivaev, I.B.; Suponitsky, K.Y.; Godovikov, I.A.; Bregadze, V.I. Synthesis of 10-methylsulfide and 10-alkylmethylsulfonium nido-carborane derivatives: B–H$\cdots\pi$ Interactions between the B–H–B hydrogen atom and alkyne group in 10-RC≡$CCH_2S(Me)$-7,8-$C_2B_9H_{11}$. *Eur. J. Inorg. Chem.* **2017**, *38*, 4436–4443. [CrossRef]
74. Anufriev, S.A.; Sivaev, I.B.; Suponitsky, K.Y.; Bregadze, V.I. Practical synthesis of 9-methylthio-7,8-nido-carborane [9-MeS-7,8-$C_2B_9H_{11}$]-. Some evidences of BH$\cdots$X hydride-halogen bonds in 9- $XCH_2(Me)S$-7,8-$C_2B_9H_{11}$ (X = Cl, Br, I). *J. Organomet. Chem.* **2017**, *849–850*, 315–323. [CrossRef]
75. Suponitsky, K.Y.; Masunov, A.E. Supramolecular step in design of nonlinear optical materials: Effect of $\pi \ldots \pi$ stacking aggregation on hyperpolarizability. *J. Chem. Phys.* **2013**, *139*, 094310. [CrossRef]

76. Bader, R.F.W. *Atoms in Molecules: A Quantum Theory*; Clarendon Press: Oxford, UK, 1990.
77. Keith, T.A. *AIMAll*; Version 15.05.18; TK Gristmill Software: Overland Park, KS, USA, 2015.
78. Espinosa, E.; Molins, E.; Lecomte, C. Hydrogen bond strengths revealed by topological analyses of experimentally observed electron densities. *Chem. Phys. Lett.* **1998**, *285*, 170–173. [CrossRef]
79. Espinosa, E.; Alkorta, I.; Rozas, I.; Elguero, J.; Molins, E. About the evaluation of the local kinetic, potential and total energy densities in closed-shell interactions. *Chem. Phys. Lett.* **2001**, *336*, 457–461. [CrossRef]
80. Suponitsky, K.Y.; Lyssenko, K.A.; Antipin, M.Y.; Aleksandrova, N.S.; Sheremetev, A.B.; Novikova, T.S. 4,4′-Bis(nitramino)azofurazan and its salts. Study of molecular and crystal structure based on X-ray and quantum chemical data. *Russ. Chem. Bull.* **2009**, *58*, 2129–2136. [CrossRef]
81. Lyssenko, K.A. Analysis of supramolecular architectures: Beyond molecular packing diagrams. *Mendeleev Commun.* **2012**, *22*, 1–7. [CrossRef]
82. Suponitsky, K.Y.; Lyssenko, K.A.; Ananyev, I.V.; Kozeev, A.M.; Sheremetev, A.B. Role of weak intermolecular interactions in the crystal structure of tetrakis-furazano[3,4-c:3′,4′-g:3″,4″-k:3‴,4‴-o][1,2,5,6,9,10,13,14]octaazacyclohexadecine and its solvates. *Cryst. Growth Des.* **2014**, *14*, 4439–4449. [CrossRef]

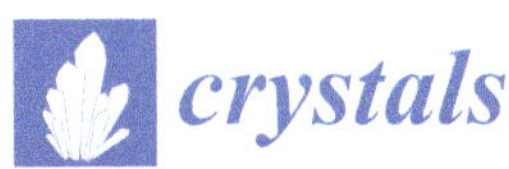 crystals

MDPI

Article

Carboranes as Lewis Acids: Tetrel Bonding in $CB_{11}H_{11}$ Carbonium Ylide

Maxime Ferrer [1], Ibon Alkorta [1], José Elguero [1] and Josep M. Oliva-Enrich [2,*]

[1] Instituto de Quimica Médica (CSIC), Juan de la Cierva, 3, E-28006 Madrid, Spain; maxime.ferrer@iqm.csic.es (M.F.); ibon@iqm.csic.es (I.A.); iqmbe17@iqm.csic.es (J.E.)
[2] Instituto de Química-Física "Rocasolano" (CSIC), Serrano, 119, E-28006 Madrid, Spain
* Correspondence: j.m.oliva@iqfr.csic.es; Tel.: +34-915619400

Abstract: High-level quantum-chemical computations (G4MP2) are carried out in the study of complexes featuring tetrel bonding between the carbon atom in the carbenoid $CB_{11}H_{11}$—obtained by hydride removal in the C-H bond of the known *closo*-monocarbadodecaborate anion $CB_{11}H_{12}{}^{(-)}$ and acting as Lewis acid (LA)—and Lewis bases (LB) of different type; the electron donor groups in the tetrel bond feature carbon, nitrogen, oxygen, fluorine, silicon, phosphorus, sulfur, and chlorine atomic centres in neutral molecules as well as anions $H^{(-)}$, $OH^{(-)}$, and $F^{(-)}$. The empty radial $2p_r$ vacant orbital on the carbon centre in $CB_{11}H_{11}$, which corresponds to the LUMO, acts as a Lewis acid or electron attractor, as shown by the molecular electrostatic potential (MEP) and electron localization function (ELF). The thermochemistry and topological analysis of the complexes {$CB_{11}H_{11}$:LB} are comprehensively analysed and classified according to shared or closed-shell interactions. ELF analysis shows that the tetrel C···X bond ranges from very polarised bonds, as in $H_{11}B_{11}C{:}F^{(-)}$ to very weak interactions as in $H_{11}B_{11}C\cdots FH$ and $H_{11}B_{11}C\cdots O{=}C{=}O$.

Keywords: Lewis acid; carborane; carbonium ylide; tetrel bond; quantum chemistry; electron density; ELF

Citation: Ferrer, M.; Alkorta, I.; Elguero, J.; Oliva-Enrich, J.M. Carboranes as Lewis Acids: Tetrel Bonding in $CB_{11}H_{11}$ Carbonium Ylide. *Crystals* **2021**, *11*, 391. https://doi.org/10.3390/cryst11040391

Academic Editor: Marina Yu. Stogniy

Received: 12 March 2021
Accepted: 2 April 2021
Published: 7 April 2021

Publisher's Note: MDPI stays neutral with regard to jurisdictional claims in published maps and institutional affiliations.

1. Introduction

The very stable $B_{12}H_{12}{}^{(2-)}$ dianion and its neutral dicarbon counterparts *ortho*-(1,2-$C_2B_{10}H_{12}$), *meta*-(1,7-$C_2B_{10}H_{12}$), and *para*-carborane (1,12-$C_2B_{10}H_{12}$) are icosahedral systems that are closely related to elemental boron. Their isoelectronic analogue, *closo*-monocarbadodecaborate anion $CB_{11}H_{12}{}^{(-)}$, first prepared in 1967 [1] and further with other synthesis methods [2,3], is similarly resistant to cage degradation, and many derivatives have been synthesized as described in the literature [4]. The stability and three-dimensional aromaticity of $CB_{11}H_{12}{}^{(-)}$ has also been explained using quantum-chemical computations [5]. Extraction of hydride $H^{(-)}$ in the C-H bond from $CB_{11}H_{12}{}^{(-)}$ leads to a carbocation ylide or carbenoid (**1**) with a vacant radial $2p_r$ orbital on the cage carbon atom as shown in Figure 1. On the other hand, reaction mechanisms of polyhedral (car)boranes and their derivatives are scarce in the literature and further research is needed in this respect [6–8]. Thus, the permethylated carbenoid analogue $CB_{11}Me_{11}$ has been postulated as a reaction intermediate during the extraction of the L substituent from L-$CB_{11}Me_{11}$ carboranes (L = $BrCH_2CH_2$ or $(CF_3)_2CHO$) by electrophiles [6,7], further reacting with arenes in the presence of $(CF_3)_2CHOH$ to generate 1-aryl-$CB_{11}Me_{11}$ products [6–8]. The methyl groups in the permethylated anion $CB_{11}Me_{12}{}^{(-)}$ have substantial $CH_3{}^{(-)}$ (methide) character according to DFT computations [6–8] and can easily bind to transition metal and main group elements.

On the other hand, in recent years, tetrel bonding—defined as an interaction between any electron donating system (ED) and a group 14 element acting as Lewis acid—has called the attention of both experimentalists [9] and theoreticians [10–12]. Here the carbon centre in (**1**) is clearly an acceptor of electrons or Lewis acid; hence, we can define a tetrel bonding interaction with an electron donor (ED) or Lewis base, as shown in Figure 1c.

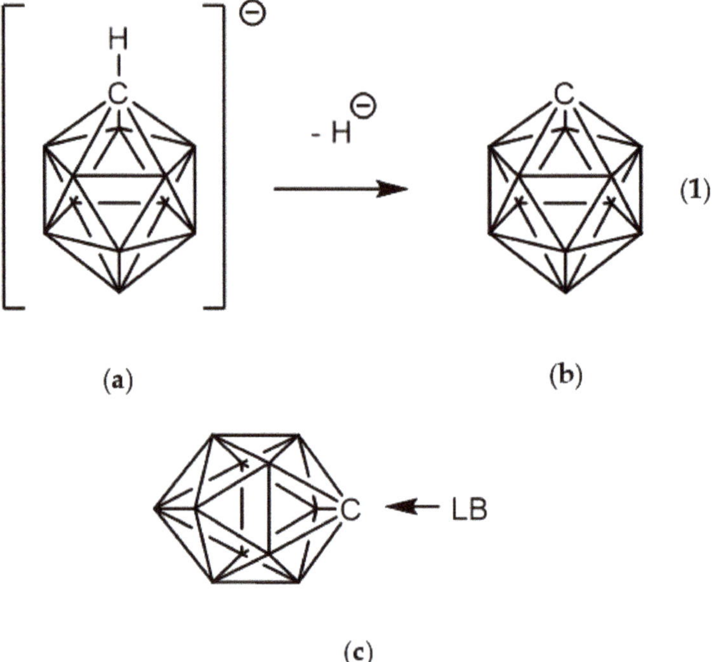

Figure 1. Removal of hydride from the C-H bond in (**a**) *closo*-monocarbadodecaborate anion $CB_{11}H_{12}^{(-)}$ leads to (**b**) carbocation ylide or carbenoid $CB_{11}H_{11}$ (**1**). (**c**) Complex formation between (**1**) and a Lewis base (LB). All vertices correspond to B-H moieties except for the carbon vertex.

The goal of this work is to study the electronic interaction between the naked carbon vertex in the carbenoid (**1**) with a series of electron donor molecules and anions leading to tetrel C-X bonds. The chosen 18 LB systems, including the anions $H^{(-)}$, $F^{(-)}$, and $OH^{(-)}$, are displayed below in Scheme 1 with the corresponding label.

$H^{(-)}$	CH_2	CF_2	C≡O	N_2	NH_3
(**2**)	(**3**)	(**4**)	(**5**)	(**6**)	(**7**)
$NH{=}CH_2$	N≡CH	$OH^{(-)}$	OH_2	$O{=}CH_2$	O=C=O
(**8**)	(**9**)	(**10**)	(**11**)	(**12**)	(**13**)
$F^{(-)}$	FH	SiH_2	PH_3	SH_2	ClH
(**14**)	(**15**)	(**16**)	(**17**)	(**18**)	(**19**)

Scheme 1. The chosen set of molecules acting as Lewis base (LB) and forming a tetrel bond with the C atom from carbenoid (**1**) according to Figure 1c.

2. Computational Methods

Electronic structure quantum-chemical computations were carried out using the G4MP2 model [13], which is a fourth-generation method available in the Gaussian16 scientific software [14]. This method combines density-functional theory [15,16] and second-order perturbation theory [17] and provides an accurate and economical method for thermochemical predictions. The G4(MP2) model works as follows: The geometries of the molecules are optimized at the B3LYP/6-31G(2df,p) level of theory, and then a series of single point energy calculations at higher levels of theory are computed. The zero-point energy, E(ZPE), is based on B3LYP/6-31G(2df,p) frequencies scaled by 0.9854, the same as in G4 theory. The first energy calculation is at the triples-augmented coupled cluster level of theory, CCSD(T), with the 6-31G(d) basis set, i.e., CCSD(T)/6-31G(d). This energy is then modified by a series of energy corrections to obtain a total energy E_0. For more details on the G4(MP2) method, the reader is referred to Reference [13]. In the particular case of the **1**:LB complexes, we computed the enthalpy and free energy differences between the complex and separated systems **1** and LB at room temperature as indication of stability of the complex. All complexes included in this work correspond to energy minimum structures, checked with frequency computations. The quantum theory of atoms-in-molecules (QTAIM) [18,19] was used in the topological analysis of the electron density of the **1**:LB complexes with the scientific software AIMAll [20]. This method is based on the analysis of the electron density ρ, its gradient $\nabla\rho$, and the corresponding Laplacian $\nabla^2\rho$. For further aspects of this methodology, the reader is referred to the above References [17,18] and Section 3.3.1 below. The electron localisation function (ELF) [21,22] was also used in the topological analysis of the complexes. The ELF is a distribution function which measures the probability of finding two electrons with the same spin, as further described in Section 3.3.2 below. The TopMod09 package [23] was used for the ELF calculations.

3. Results

3.1. Geometries of Complexes (1:n), n = 2–19

In Figure 2a,b we display the G4MP2 optimized geometries of $CB_{11}H_{12}^{(-)}$ with C_{5v} symmetry—the (**1**:**2**) complex and the carbonium ylide $CB_{11}H_{11}$ (**1**), with the different tetrel complexes (**1**:***n***), ***n*** = **2–19** and structural parameters when necessary, in order to highlight the atomic rearrangements undergone due to the complexation process. The loss of $H^{(-)}$ in the C-H leads also to a structure with C_{5v} symmetry—with a geometrical change which involves a considerable flattening of the CB_5 pentagonal pyramid with expansion of the corresponding B_5 pentagon, since there is an increase of the B-B bond distance of Δ = +0.022 Å. As we proceed down the cage from the top (C atom), the B-B bond differences are +0.022 Å, +0.022 Å, and −0.015 Å. Quite noticeable is the shortening of the apical intracage C$\cdots$B distance ($\Delta\sim-0.3$ Å). The B-H bond distances hardly change at all, with a very slight shortening upon loss of $H^{(-)}$ with Δ = −0.007 Å, −0.008 Å, and −0.001 Å, from top to bottom, respectively. If we take the C and B cage nuclei as point charges and define a distorted C_{5v} icosahedron, the corresponding volumes are $V(CB_{11}H_{12}^{(-)})$ = 12.03 Å^3 and $V(CB_{11}H_{11})$ = 11.90 Å^3, and therefore there is a shrinkage of the cage by ΔV = −0.13 Å^3 (1%). In summary, the extraction of hydride in the C-H bond from $CB_{11}H_{12}^{(-)}$ implies a minor change in the cage volume with a flattening of the top CB_5 pentagonal pyramid and minor changes as we proceed down the cage from the top C atom. In Figure 2c–s, we display the optimised geometries for the remaining complexes with the coordinates gathered in the Supplementary Material (SI, Tables S1–S10). The shortest and longest C$\cdots$X tetrel interactions correspond to the original anion $CB_{11}H_{12}^{(-)}$ or complex (**1**:**2**) and the $CB_{11}H_{11}\cdots$O=C=O tetrel complex (**1**:**13**), respectively. In the latter case, the interaction is clearly non-covalent in origin with d(C$\cdots$O) = 2.693 Å, as will be discussed later on. We should also emphasize the C$\cdots$X interaction of the CH_2 and SiH_2 complexes (**1**:**3**) and (**1**:**16**), respectively, with the LB groups tilted from the C_5 axis of rotation. In all other systems, including the CF_2 complex (**1**:**4**), the C$\cdots$X bond is aligned with the C_5 axis of rotation.

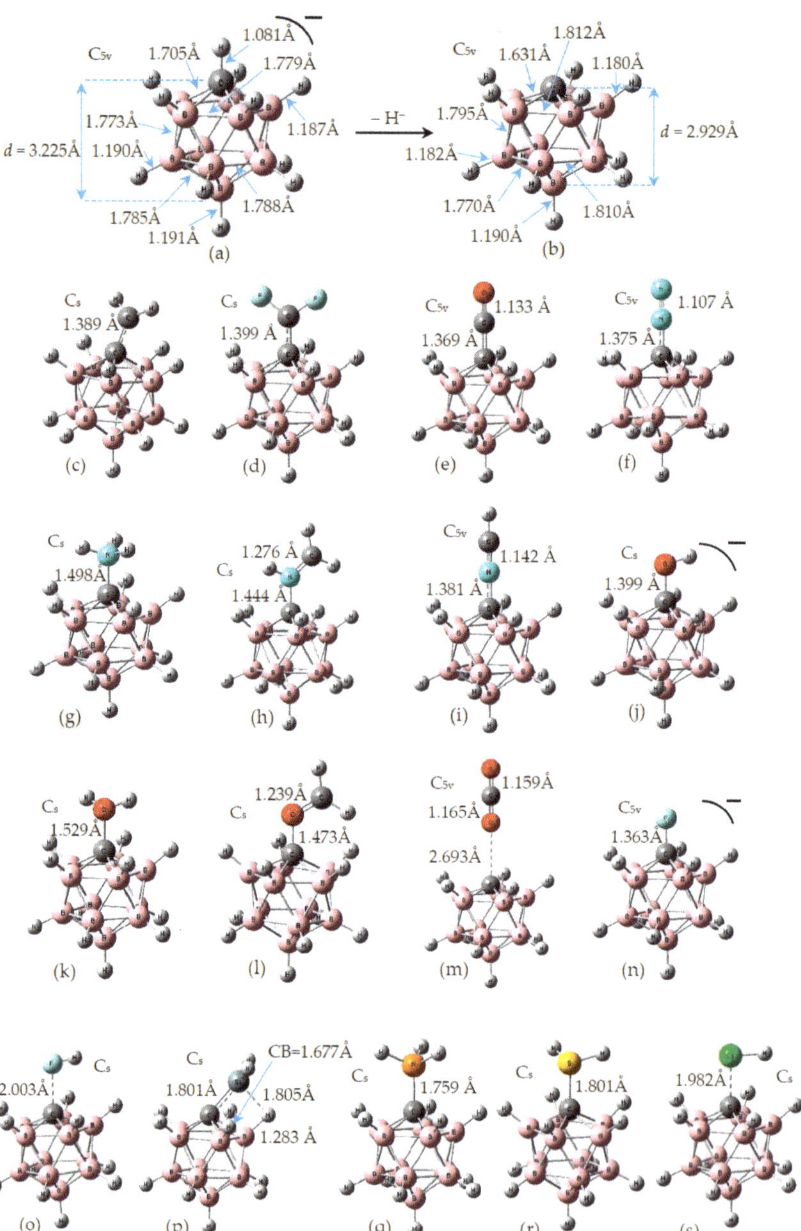

Figure 2. Structures of the G4MP2 optimized geometries for the 18 tetrel complexes (**1**:***n***)—with ***n*** = **2–19**—considered in this work, following Scheme 1: (**a**) The known anion $CB_{11}H_{12}^{(-)}$ corresponding to complex (**1**:**2**), (**b**) carbenoid $CB_{11}H_{11}$ (**1**), (**c**) (**1**:**3**), (**d**) (**1**:**4**), (**e**) (**1**:**5**), (**f**) (**1**:**6**), (**g**) (**1**:**7**), (**h**) (**1**:**8**), (**i**) (**1**:**9**), (**j**) (**1**:**10**), (**k**) (**1**:**11**), (**l**) (**1**:**12**), (**m**) (**1**:**13**), (**n**) (**1**:**14**), (**o**) (**1**:**15**), (**p**) (**1**:**16**), (**q**) (**1**:**17**), (**r**) (**1**:**18**), and (**s**) (**1**:**19**).

In Figure 3, we display the d(C$\cdots$X) distances in the tetrel bonding complexes, ordered from shortest to longest. Clearly, we can classify five groups according to the C$\cdots$X distances, in increasing order: (i) The original anion $CB_{11}H_{12}^{(-)}$ or (**1**:**2**) complex; (ii) complexes with d~1.4–1.5 Å including complexes (**1:k$_2$**), with k$_2$ = (3–12, 14); (iii) complexes with d~1.8 Å, including complexes (**1:k$_3$**), with k$_3$ = 16–18; (iv) complexes with d~2.0 Å, including complexes (**1:15**) and (**1:19**); and finally (v) the (**1:13**) complex with d~2.7 Å.

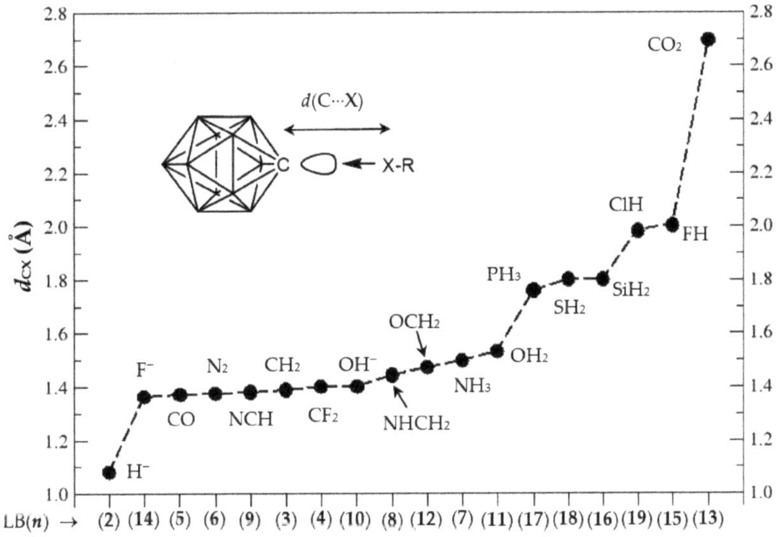

Figure 3. C· · · X distances d_{CX} (Å) in the tetrel complexes (**1:*n***), ***n*** **= 2–19**, from Figure 2, in increasing order; x axis corresponds to Lewis base (LB) *n* and y axis to d_{CX} distances (Å), respectively.

*3.2. Thermochemistry of Complexes (**1:n**), **n = 2–19***

In this subsection, we predict the ΔH and ΔG of the tetrel bonding complexes (**1:*n***), ***n*** **= 2–19**. In Table 1, we gather the computed enthalpies and free energies at the G4MP2 level of theory.

Table 1. Enthalpy (ΔH) and free energy (ΔG) of formation for complexes (**1:*n***), ***n*** **= 2–19**, in kJ·mol^{-1}. LB: Lewis base.

	n = 2	3	4	5	6	7	8	9	10
LB	$H^{(-)}$	CH_2	CF_2	C≡O	N_2	NH_3	NH=CH$_2$	N≡CH	$OH^{(-)}$
ΔH	−858.6	−504.9	−326.2	−211.1	−50.5	−268.6	−294.6	−170.6	−659.3
ΔG	−822.3	−457.7	−279.7	−162.9	−2.8	−226.8	−242.7	−120.8	−618.0

	11	12	13	14	15	16	17	18	19
LB	OH_2	O=CH$_2$	O=C=O	$F^{(-)}$	FH	SiH_2	PH_3	SH_2	ClH
ΔH	−116.2	−139.8	−14.3	−571.5	−0.7	−418.0	−280.9	−186.1	−47.6
ΔG	−72.1	−87.9	25.7	−529.7	31.3	−366.8	−238.1	−140.9	−8.9

The free energy of formation for complexes (**1:*n***) is always negative except for (**1:13**) and (**1:15**) complexes, namely the O=C=O and FH complexes, respectively. Small negative values (|ΔG| < 10 kJ·mol^{-1}) are obtained for complexes (**1:6**) and (**1:19**) with Lewis bases N_2 and ClH, respectively. Therefore, all complexes with negative ΔG should be formed at room temperature spontaneously, provided an isolated Lewis acid (**1**) approaches an isolated Lewis base. On the other hand, the enthalpies of formation are negative for all complexes, an indication that the bond energies of a given complex (**1:*n***) have a lower value than the bond energies of separated systems (**1**) and (***n***). In order to better visualize the similarities and differences of the thermochemical aspects of complexes (**1**:***n***), we plot ΔG and ΔH vs. ***n*** in increasing order of each state function.

As shown in Figure 4 from left to right in the abscissa, the ΔG (black) and ΔH (blue) in complex formation follow the same order as function of Lewis base number except for ClH (**1**:**19**) and N_2 (**1**:**6**), where the order is inverted in the ΔH tendency as compared to ΔG. Hence, the formation of anionic complexes are the most energetic and favourable ones in the order (**1**:**2**), (**1**:**10**), (**1**:**14**) corresponding to Lewis bases $H^{(-)}$, $OH^{(-)}$, and $F^{(-)}$, respectively; then follow complexes (**1**:**3**), (**1**:**16**), and (**1**:**4**) corresponding to Lewis bases CH_2, SiH_2 and CF_2, respectively, namely the carbene series. A plateau with complexes (**1**:**8**), (**1**:**17**), and (**1**:**7**) follows with Lewis bases $NH{=}CH_2$, PH_3, and NH_3, respectively. A smaller (positive) slope of ΔG/ΔH vs. *n* appears with complexes (**1**:**5**), (**1**:**18**), (**1**:**9**), (**1**:**12**), and (**1**:**11**) always in increasing order, which correspond to Lewis bases C≡O, SH_2, N≡CH, $O{=}CH_2$, and OH_2, respectively. The weakest bound complexes with ΔG < 0 correspond to (**1**:**19**) and (**1**:**6**) with Lewis bases ClH and N_2, respectively. Finally, complexes (**1**:**13**) and (**1**:**15**) with Lewis bases O=C=O and FH, respectively, show a predicted quantum-chemical value of ΔG > 0, and therefore one should not expect a spontaneous formation of these complexes at room temperature. It is noteworthy to mention the tiny value ΔH(**1**:**15**) = -0.7 kJ·mol^{-1} for FH attachment to (**1**); this number is within the accuracy of the method and therefore a heat of formation for complex (**1**:**15**) or the bond energy on both sides of the equation remains unaltered.

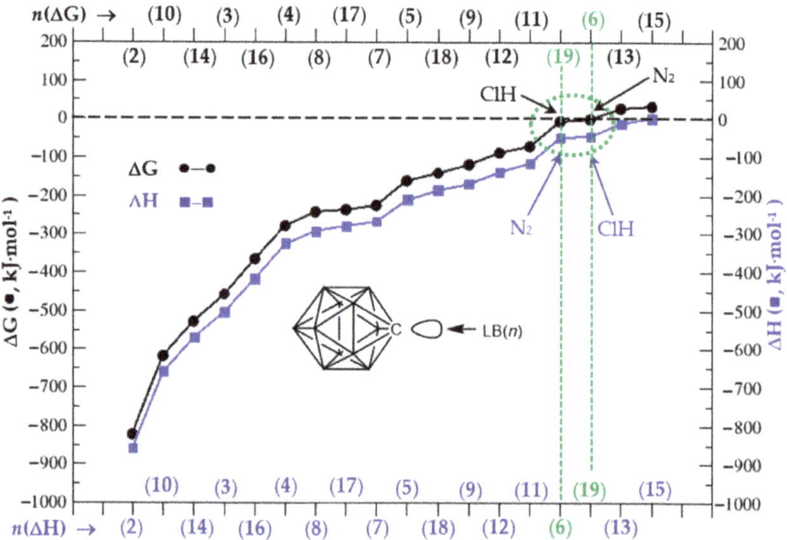

Figure 4. ΔG and ΔH vs. Lewis base ***n*** in respective increasing order, all in kJ·mol^{-1}.

3.3. *Electronic Structure of Complexes (**1**:**n**), **n** = 2–19*

In Figure 5, we show for (**1**) the molecular electrostatic potential (MEP) and the electron localization function (ELF). These electronic structure features are computed using the optimized geometry of the system with the G4MP2 method—B3LYP/6-31G(2df,p) model chemistry for structure optimization. As noticed in Figure 5a, the shape of the MEP and the corresponding π-hole just on top of the C ylide centre shows the electron-attraction nature of this region of the molecule. In the ELF from Figure 5b, we show disynaptic V(B,H) yellow basins corresponding to the B-H bonds; the ELF distribution around the CB_{11} icosahedral cage can be partitioned into green disynaptic and trisynaptic basins, as we will describe below in Section 3.3.2.

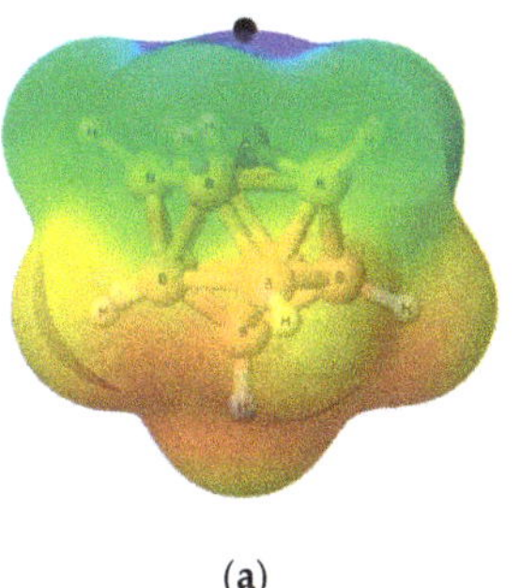

(a)

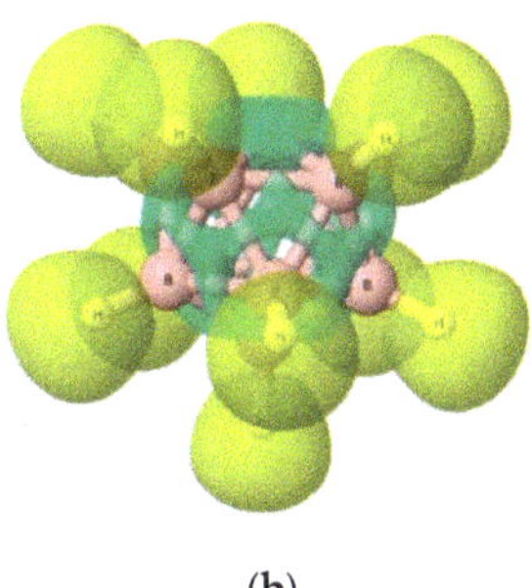

(b)

Figure 5. Electronic structure of carbonium ylide (**1**) $CB_{11}H_{11}$: (**a**) Molecular electrostatic potential V(**r**). Red colour for V(**r**) < −0.015 au, Blue colour for V(**r**) > 0.03 au. The black dot indicates the localization of the π-hole (0.061 au), and (**b**) Electron Localization Function (ELF) with an isosurface of ELF = 0.75. Computations with the G4MP2 level of theory.

The molecular electrostatic potential (MEP) is the potential energy of a proton at a particular location near a molecule. Negative electrostatic potential corresponds to an attraction of the proton by the concentrated electron density in the molecules. The MEP of (**1**)—Figure 5b—shows that the potential energy of a proton is most positive above the C atom with a π-hole of +0.061 au, hence a repulsive region for a proton approaching (**1**), or electron acceptor region. The MEP is smoothly changing from positive to negative values of the potential energy as the proton moves from the C atom down to the B skeleton cage region. A proton would then be attached more favourably to the lower region of the carbonium ylide (**1**). In other words, Lewis bases, electron donors, and nucleophiles should then tend to bind through the C atom of the ylide, hence the study of the tetrel bonding in the complexes (**1**:***n***).

3.3.1. Atoms-in-Molecules (AIM) Topological Analysis of Complexes (1:*n*), *n* = 2–19

The Quantum Theory of Atoms in Molecules (QTAIM) [18,19] is a useful tool for analysing the electronic structure of a polyatomic many-electron system, with the electron density $\rho(\mathbf{r})$ as the central function. The topological properties of $\rho(\mathbf{r})$ are analysed with the gradient of $\nabla\rho(\mathbf{r})$, the Laplacian of $\rho(\mathbf{r})$, $\nabla^2\rho(\mathbf{r})$, and the eigenvalues of the Hessian matrix of the electron density λ_1, λ_2, λ_3. The critical points are those with $\vec{\nabla}\rho = \vec{0}$ and a bond critical point (BCP) has $\lambda_3 > 0$ associated with the bond path direction, and $\lambda_1 < 0$, $\lambda_2 < 0$ the two latter associated to two directions where $\nabla^2\rho$ is a maximum; the BCP (−,−,+) appears at the intersection of the bond path with the interatomic surface S. Other critical points are classified according to the signs of λ_i: Nuclei positions with (−, −, −); ring critical points with (−,+,+); cage critical points with (+,+,+). We should also introduce the local electron kinetic (G > 0), potential (V < 0), and total (H) energy densities, with H = G + V, also useful parameters at the BCP for the description of the type of bonding interaction between atoms in a many-electron system [24]. In the SI (Table S11), we provide the computed values of $\rho(\mathbf{r})$, $\nabla\rho(\mathbf{r})$, $\nabla^2\rho(\mathbf{r})$, G, V, and H for the BCP found between the X atom of the Lewis base in contact with the C ylide centre in (**1**), for all complexes (**1**:***n***), ***n*** = **2–19**.

In Figure 6a, we plot the electron density at the BCP for the C···X interaction vs. *d*(CX) distance. The largest values of ρ_{BCP} correspond to CH_2 ($\rho_{BCP}(CH_2) = 0.32\ e/a_0^3$), CF_2, and CO, followed by $H^{(-)}$, $OH^{(-)}$, $NHCH_2$, N_2, and $F^{(-)}$. Another group follows with lower values, NH_3, OCH_2, PH_3, OH_2, SH_2, and further down, SiH_2 and ClH with similar values. Finally, the lowest ρ_{BCP} correspond to FH and CO_2, the latter with $\rho_{BCP}(CO_2) = 0.01\ e/a_0^3$. We should emphasize that the ratio $\rho_{BCP,max}(CH_2)/\rho_{BCP,min}(CO_2) = 32$ gives an idea of the topological differences in these BCPs. Given the different type of C···X interactions in the complexes, the ρ_{BCP} vs. *d*(CX) can be fit to an approximate negative exponential curve with $\rho_{BCP}(d_{CX}) = a + b\cdot\exp(-c\cdot d_{CX})$, with $a = -0.022$, $b = +3.222$, and $c = -1.751$, and a correlation factor of $R^2 = 0.99$ for closed-shell interacting complexes: CO_2, FH, SiH_2, N_2, and NCH. This curve is displayed in the SI (Figure S1). In general, very good correlations appear if we fix the two interacting atoms both belonging to the same row of the Periodic Table [25–27].

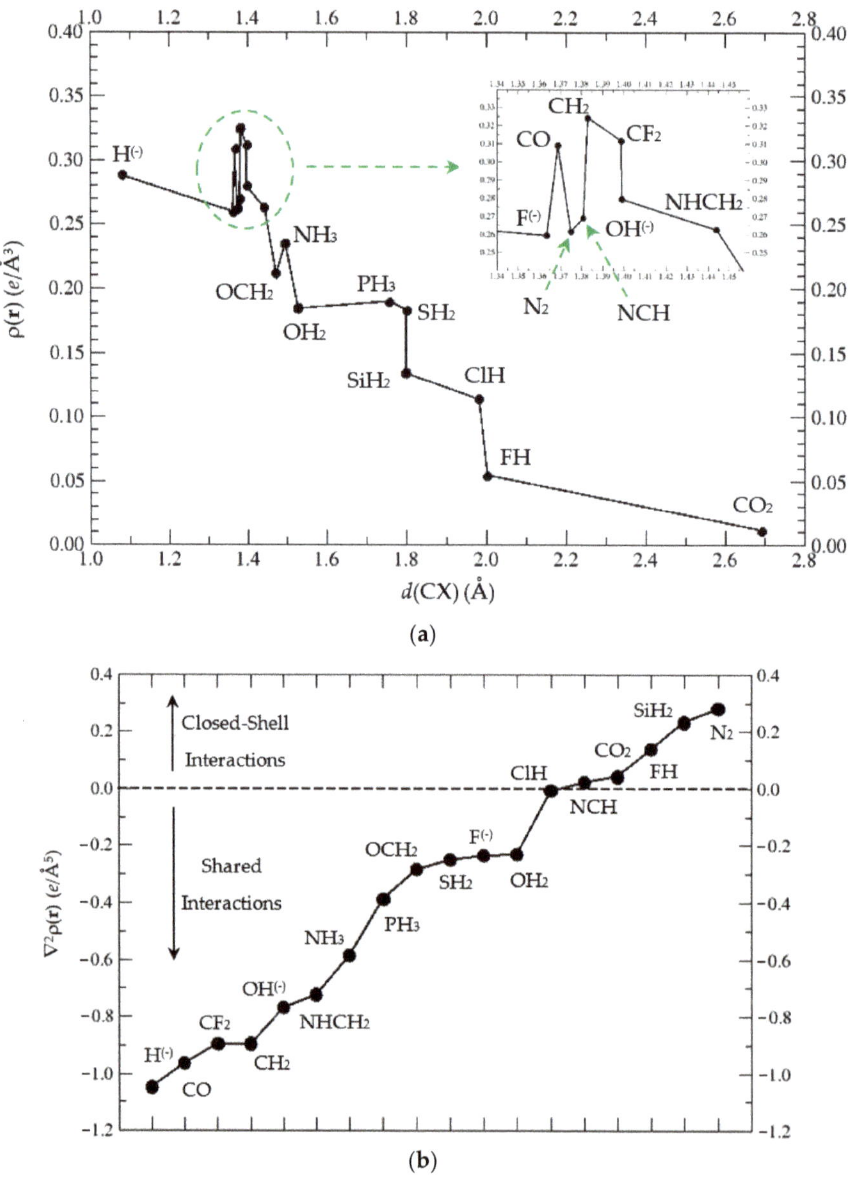

Figure 6. *Cont.*

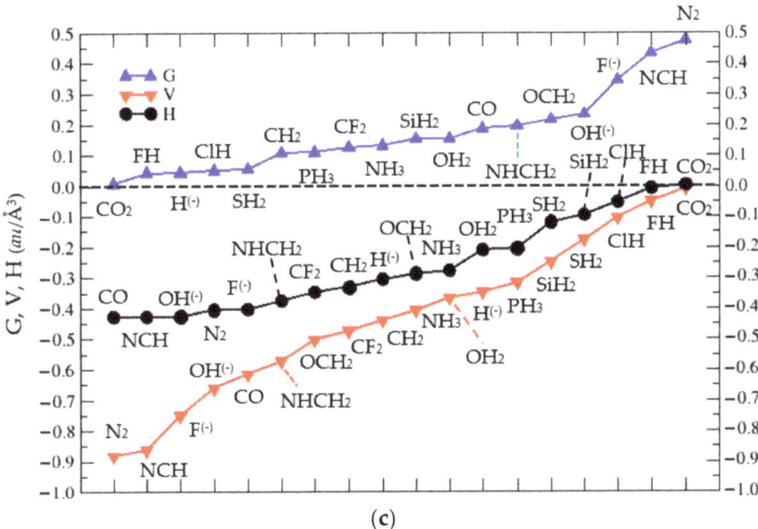

Figure 6. **(a).** $\rho(\mathbf{r})$ at the BCP of the C$\cdots$X interaction in complexes (**1**:$\boldsymbol{n}$) vs. d(CX), with $\boldsymbol{n}$ = **2–19**. We label each point with the corresponding LB. **(b)** $\nabla^2\rho(\mathbf{r})$ at the C$\cdots$X BCP for complexes (**1**:$\boldsymbol{n}$), $\boldsymbol{n}$ = **2–19**. **(c)** Plot of G (▲), V (▼), and H (•) vs. Lewis base LB($\boldsymbol{n}$) in increasing order of G, V, and H, respectively, at the Bond Critical Point (BCP) in the C$\cdots$X interaction of complexes (**1**:$\boldsymbol{n}$), $\boldsymbol{n}$ = **2–19**, as described in Scheme 1.

In order to estimate the type of interaction we need to go beyond the electron density at the BCP and analyse the second derivative, the Laplacian $\nabla^2\rho$, and the kinetic, potential, and total energy, G, V, and H respectively, of the BCPs in complexes (**1**:$\boldsymbol{n}$). In Figure 6b, the Laplacian is plotted vs. LB($\boldsymbol{n}$) in increasing order. Clearly, we can distinguish the shared interactions for $\nabla^2\rho < 0$ in the lower left corner and closed-shell interactions for $\nabla^2\rho > 0$ in the upper right corner of Figure 6b. The two-electron sharing in complexes with $H^{(-)}$, CO, CF_2, and CH_2 is large, and it is diminished up to OH_2. For the complex with HCl, $\nabla^2\rho = -0.0067\ e/\text{Å}^5$, namely in the limit between shared and closed-shell interactions. For positive Laplacians, in increasing order, the LB in the (**1**:$\boldsymbol{n}$) complexes correspond to: NCH, CO_2, FH, SiH_2, and N_2; in these systems, the closed-shell interactions are important.

A further analysis of the BCP in the C$\cdots$X interactions of the (**1**:$\boldsymbol{n}$) complexes can be found in the values of G, V, and H—with H = G + V being the total energy—as displayed in Figure 6c. The kinetic energy G is associated with repulsion in the bonding region, and the local potential energy density or local virial field V is a measure of the average effective potential field experienced by a single electron in a many-particle system. Thus, according to Figure 6c, the G and V profiles are inverted for N_2, NCH, $F^{(-)}$, and $OH^{(-)}$, but due to the nature of different nuclei in the C-X interactions, this is not always the case, as seen when we follow the profiles as function of LB($\boldsymbol{n}$).

3.3.2. Electron Localisation Function (ELF) Analysis of Complexes (1:*n*), *n* = 2–19

We should emphasize that ELF is a function which reports the probability of finding an electron pair with opposite spins in a region of space. Using a certain isovalue, we are able to define regions of space, basins, with a certain probability to find an electron pair. For example, in the plots of the ELF, we used an isovalue of 0.83; in other words, we plot regions of space where we have a high probability to find a pair of electrons. Once the basins are defined, we can integrate the electronic density into those basins, which are the values reported above in Table 2 and correspond to the number of electrons in that basin. In ELF analysis, the partition of space is not based on the electron density, as in AIM, but on the ELF probability function. In order to better understand from the electronic structure point of view the tetrel bonding in the (**1:*n***) complexes, we further computed the electron localisation function (ELF) [21,22,28], a measure of the likelihood of finding an electron in the neighborhood space of a reference electron located at a given point and with the same spin; therefore, ELF is a measure of the Pauli repulsion or exchange interaction [29,30]. The ELF for the carbonium ylidene $CB_{11}H_{11}$ (**1**) is shown in Figure 4. ELF values ranges from zero to one (normalized and without units). In the SI file we provide the ELF for all complexes (**1:*n***) not shown here (Table S12), and below we have selected four cases with short, medium, long, and very long C··· X distances, according to Figure 3 above: (i) LB = $H^{(-)}$, complex (**1:2**), (ii) LB = N_2, complex (**1:6**), (iii) LB = PH_3, complex (**1:17**), and (iv) LB = CO_2, complex (**1:13**). In Table 2, we gather the ELF function for these four complexes.

Table 2. Electron localisation function (ELF) (isovalue 0.83 au) for complexes $H_{11}B_{11}C{:}H^{(-)} \rightarrow$ (**1:2**), $H_{11}B_{11}C{:}N{\equiv}N \rightarrow$ (**1:6**), $H_{11}B_{11}C{:}PH_3 \rightarrow$ (**1:17**), and $H_{11}B_{11}C{:}O{=}C{=}O \rightarrow$ (**1:13**). Basin labels are depicted for each complex. Population of ELF disynaptic basins V(C, X) in bold.

$H^{(-)}$	N≡N	PH_3	CO_2
11 C(B) = 2.07	11 C(B) = 2.06	11 C(B) = 2.07	11 C(B) = 2.07
1 C(C) = 2.11	1 C(C) = 2.06	1 C(C) = 2.07	2 C(C) = 2.07
11 V(B,H) = 2.05	2 C(N) = 2.07	1 C(P) = 9.89	2 C(O) = 2.13
10 V(B,B,B) = 0.81	11 V(B,H) = 2.05	11 V(B,H) = 2.05	11 V(B,H) = 2.03
15 V(B,B) = 0.76	1 V(N,N) = 4.01	3 V(P,H) = 2.05	1 V(C2,O2) = 2.26
5 V(C,B) = 1.01	5 V(B,B) = 0.46	5 V(C,B) = 1.01	1 V(C2,O1) = 2.51
1 V(C,H) = 2.05	5 V(B,B,B) = 2.43	**1 V(C,P) = 2.21**	5 V(C,B) = 1.20
	5 V(B,B,B) = 0.97	5 V(B,B) = 0.51	15 V(B,B) = 0.54
	5 V(C,B) = 1.02	5 V(B,B,B) = 2.44	7 V(B,B,B) = 1.08
	1 V(C,N2) = 2.62	5 V(B,B,B) = 0.91	3 V(C,B,B) = 1.08
	1 V(N1) = 3.51		1 V(O2) = 5.64
			1 V(O1) = 3.44
			1 V(O1) = 1.82

Below each ELF function of a given complex (**1:*n***), we also report the function value and average population for the different types of basins. A threshold of 0.2 electrons is considered as to include or not a basin in a group. Below each ELF function of a given complex (**1:*n***), we report the population of the different basins. In order to avoid dealing with a long list of populations and after observing that basins involving the same elements have similar populations, we decided to report only for each type of basins the average population. A threshold of 0.2 electrons was chosen to decide if two basins belong to the same group or not. For instance, if we consider basins $V(B_1,B_2)$ and $V(B_1,B_3)$ with populations of 0.8 and 1.5 electrons, respectively, they belong to different groups. In bold letters, we report the value of the disynaptic basin corresponding to the tetrel C··· X interaction.

In Table 2 we use the following notation:

- C: core basin
- V(X): monosynaptic basin, which can be associated to a lone pair
- V(X,X): disynaptic basin
- V(X,X,X): trisynaptic basin

- 5 V(B,B) = 0.42: There are 5 disynaptic basins involving two boron atoms with an average population of 0.42 electrons.

In the ELF representation, the following colours are used:

- Blue: core basin
- Red: monosynaptic basin
- Grey: polysynaptic basin
- Beige: V(X,H) basin
- Atoms: Boron (green), Carbon (black), Hydrogen (silver), Oxygen (red), and Phosphorus (tan).

Thus, according to Table 2, in the complex (**1:2**), the existing anion $CB_{11}H_{12}{}^{(-)}$, the 11 core electrons from the boron cage, the $1s^2$(B) ones, are gathered in the C(B) core basins, which have an average population of 2.07 electrons; the same description applies for the single C atom and the C(C) = 2.11 basin. The 11 B-H bonds on each non-naked B vertex of the icosahedron correspond to the 11 V(B,H) = 2.05, basically a two-electron covalent B-H bond. Then the distribution of the remaining valence cage electrons (corresponding to 2*s* and 2*p* electrons from B and C, plus the surplus electron or negative charge of the anion) are distributed in the 10 V(B,B,B) trisynaptic basins with an average population of 0.81 electrons, the 15 V(B,B) disynaptic basins with a population of 0.76 electrons, and the 5 V(C,B) disynaptic basins with ~1 electron in them. The V(C,H) disynaptic basin, with a population of 2.05, corresponds to the C···X = C-H bond in (**1:2**), a two-centre two-electron bond. Addition of the values of all basins leads to the number of electrons in $CB_{11}H_{12}{}^{(-)}$: 74.

As reported in Table 2, the C···X interaction in the selected complexes can be described by the presence or absence of V(C,X) valence basins and its population. For the complexes (**1:6**) and (**1:17**), these values are $V_{(1:6)}$(C,N) = 2.62 and $V_{(1:17)}$(C,P) = 2.21, respectively. Therefore, ELF describes the C···X for the N_2 complex as a bond, with a multiplicity close to 1.5, between the C(ylide) and N nuclei and for the PH_3 complex a C(ylide)P single bond, with additional 0.2 electrons. As regard to the (**1:13**) complex with CO_2, the ELF does not localize a basin between the C(ylide) and the O=C=O molecule; the absence of ELF basins indicate that electron pairs are not shared, and therefore, the interaction is not covalent. However, other interactions such as ionic or non-covalent are possible even in the absence of ELF basins. The lone pairs from N_2 and CO_2 appear as red monosynaptic basins, as displayed in Table 2.

4. Discussion

The presence of a filled or empty lone pair on the C atom in the known anion $CB_{11}H_{12}{}^{(-)}$, complex (**1:2**), depends on whether we remove a proton or a hydride from the C-H bond, leading to a dianion $[CB_{11}H_{11}]^{(2-)}$ (**1b**) or a carbonium ylide $CB_{11}H_{11}$ (**1**), respectively; the latter process is shown in Figure 1. The tetrel complexes (**1:*n***) presented in the previous section show a rich variety of thermochemical and electronic structure features with tetrel C···X interactions from different nuclei: X = {H, C, N, O, F, Si, P, Cl}. The C(ylide) centre in (**1**) confers to this particular molecule with a Lewis acid (LA) character, hence the tetrel denomination. The strength for electronic attachment in (**1**) is given by the computed free energy of formation (**1**) + (***n***) → (**1:*n***). The strongest complexes correspond to those formed with anions $H^{(-)}$, $OH^{(-)}$, and $F^{(-)}$, and the weakest complexes to those formed with FH, CO_2, N_2, and ClH. The C···X distance varies considerably in all complexes, ranging from 1.081 Å for (**1:2**), LB = $H^{(-)}$, to 2.694 Å for (**1:13**), LB = CO_2. The complex strength is not related to the C···X distance; namely, complexes with similar C···X distances may have different free energy of formation, e.g., the free energy of formation for complexes (**1:14**) LB = $F^{(-)}$ and (**1:6**) LB = N_2 is -530 kJ·mol^{-1} and -3 kJ·mol^{-1}, respectively, with very similar d(C-X) distances, 1.364 Å and 1.375 Å.

Examples of recent related systems is the 3D analogue of phenyllithium, the lithiacarborane $CB_{11}H_{11}$:$Li^{(-)}$, studied in solution as a solid and by quantum-chemical computations [31]. Indeed, $Li^{(-)}$ is a very poor Lewis base but certainly attaches to (**1**), as recently shown, and defined as the lithiated mono-anion $[Li{-}CB_{11}H_{11}]^{(-)}$. On the other hand, this process can also be seen as a carborane dianion $[CB_{11}H_{11}]^{(2-)}$—a very reactive species—attached to $Li^{(+)}$, as described in Reference [31]. Table 8-1 from the book by Grimes, *Carboranes* [4], reports hundreds of compounds derived from $CB_{11}H_{12}{}^{(-)}$, and therefore this is a rich field not only from a synthetic point of view but also for studying the electronic structure of tetrel C· · · X bonds in these compounds, and especially if the isolated tetrel complexes (**1:*n***) could ever be synthesized, taking into account that this work is purely theoretical with predictive quantum-chemical computations.

The electronic structure of the complexes has been analysed thoroughly with AIM and ELF methods, showing the C· · · X sharing and closed-shell interactions in the complexes according to the values of the Laplacian of the electron density. In Table 3, we gather the ELF values for disynaptic basins V(C, X) in the C· · · X region showing values of ELF: we can find very polarised C-F bonds in (1:14)—only one electron in the C· · · X region—single C-X bonds for $H^{(-)}$ and $NH{=}CH_2$ and intermediate cases, such as in complex (1:5) with a 1.5 multiplicity C-C bond for the CO complex. No V(C,X) disynaptic basins are found for CO_2 and FH, an indication of the poor electron-donating ability of these Lewis bases (LB) with indeed long *d*(C-X) distances and positive free energies of formation $\Delta G > 0$, hence confirming the unlikely formation of these two complexes.

Table 3. Population of ELF disynaptic basins V(C, X) in tetrel complexes (**1:*n***), ***n* = 2–19**, describing the C· · · X interaction. LB = Lewis base.

n	LB	V(C, X)	*n*	LB	V(C, X)
2	$H^{(-)}$	2.05	11	OH_2	1.56
3	CH_2	2.53	12	$O{=}CH_2$	1.65
4	CF_2	2.71	13	O=C=O	-
5	C≡O	2.78	14	$F^{(-)}$	0.99
6	N≡N	2.62	15	FH	-
7	NH_3	1.76	16	SiH_2	2.40
8	$NH{=}CH_2$	2.02	17	PH_3	2.21
9	N≡CH	2.34	18	SH_2	1.85
10	$OH^{(-)}$	1.32	19	ClH	1.11

According to the Cambridge structural database(CSD) [32], several tetrel complexes derived from (1) have been characterised [33–39] where the C(ylide) centre interacts with a nitrogen atom from neutral aminoderivatives including pyridine. These structures are shown in the SI file as Table S13. The shortest C(ylide)· · · N distance, *d*(C· · · N) = 1.477 Å, corresponds to the pyridine complex 1-(4-methoxypyridinium)-1-carba-*closo*-dodecaborane [33]. The longest C(ylide)· · · N distance, *d*(C· · · N) = 1.554 Å, corresponds to the complex 12-iodo-1-(4-pentylquinuclidine)-1-carba-*closo*-dodecaborane [34]. There is a tetrel complex of (**1**) with NH_3, 1-amino-2-fluorocarba-*closo*-dodecaborane [35], where one B-H vertex hydrogen atom on position 2 has been substituted by a fluorine atom with *d*(C· · · N) = 1.486 Å. Our (**1:7**) tetrel complex $H_{11}B_{11}C \leftarrow{:}NH_3$ has a predicted *d*(C· · · N) = 1.498 Å according to the G4MP2 computational model.

5. Conclusions

The results presented in this work show that by means of quantum-chemical computations we should expect the formation of tetrel complexes between the icosahedral carbonium ylide $CB_{11}H_{11}$—derived from extraction of $H^{(-)}$ in the known anion $CB_{11}H_{12}{}^{(-)}$—and a set of simple molecules and anions. The driving force of formation for these complexes can be accounted for from thermochemical quantum-chemical computations using statistical mechanics implemented in the scientific software Gaussian16 [14], and the results indicate that all the complexes should be formed with the exception of the FH and CO_2 molecules, with N_2 and ClH complexes with indeed very low, though negative, free energies of formation.

The tetrel C···X interactions in all complexes have been thoroughly studied by means of AIM and ELF methods, hence defining the type of bond and interaction, ranging from very polarised bonds, with one electron in the C···X moiety, to intermediate cases as in the carbenes CH_2 and CF_2 and silane SiH_2, with one and a half electrons in the C···X region.

The existence of known tetrel complexes of the carbonium ylide $CB_{11}H_{11}$ with amino derivatives, including pyridine, opens the door toward further experimental and theoretical studies in the electronic structure of unusual bonds and interactions between C(ylide) centres in carboranes and other atoms.

We hope that the results from this work can be used for the isolation of reactive species, such as the recently found dianion derived from proton extraction in the well-known carborane anion $CB_{11}H_{12}^{(-)}$, a key molecule in the description of 3D aromaticity within boron chemistry.

Supplementary Materials: The following are available online at https://www.mdpi.com/article/10.3390/cryst11040391/s1, Tables S1–S10. G4MP2 optimised geometries of complexes (**1**:***n***). Table S11. AIM data for complexes (**1**:***n***). Table S12. ELF data for complexes (**1**:***n***) not displayed in the main text.

Author Contributions: Writing-original draft preparation, computations, and data curation: J.M.O.-E., M.F., I.A., and J.E. All authors have read and agreed to the published version of the manuscript.

Funding: This research was funded by Spanish MICINN, grant number CTQ2018-094644-B-C22 and Comunidad de Madrid, grant number P2018/EMT-4329 AIRTEC-CM.

Data Availability Statement: Not applicable.

Conflicts of Interest: The authors declare no conflict of interest.

References

1. Knoth, W.H. 1-$B_9H_9CH^-$ and $B_{11}H_{11}CH^-$. *J. Am. Chem. Soc.* **1967**, *89*, 1274–1275. [CrossRef]
2. Plešek, J.; Jelínek, T.; Drdáková, E.; Heřmánek, S.; Štíbr, B. A convenient preparation of 1-$CB_{11}H_{12}^-$ and its C-amino derivatives. *Collect. Czechoslov. Chem. Commun.* **1984**, *49*, 1559–1562. [CrossRef]
3. Franken, A.; King, B.T.; Rudolph, J.; Rao, P.; Noll, B.C.; Michl, J. Preparation of [*closo*-$CB_{11}H_{12}$]$^-$ by dichlorocarbene insertion into [*nido*-$B_{11}H_{14}$]. *Collect. Czechoslov. Chem. Commun.* **2001**, *66*, 1238–1249. [CrossRef]
4. Grimes, R.N. *Carboranes*, 3rd ed.; Academic Press: Cambridge, MA, USA, 2016.
5. Schleyer, P.v.R.; Najafian, K. Stability and three-dimensional aromaticity of *closo*-monocarbaborane anions, $CB_{n\text{-}1}H_n^-$,and closo-dicarboranes, $C_2B_{n\text{-}2}H_n$. *Inorg. Chem.* **1998**, *37*, 3454–3470. [CrossRef] [PubMed]
6. Michl, J. Chemistry of the three-dimensionally aromatic CB_{11} cage. *Pure Appl. Chem.* **2008**, *80*, 429–446. [CrossRef]
7. Vyakaranam, K.; Körbe, S.; Divišová, H.; Michl, J. A new type of intermediate, $C^+(BCH_3)_{11}^- \leftrightarrow C(BCH_3)_{11}$, in a Grob fragmentation coupled with intramolecular hydride transfer. A nonclassical carbocation ylide or a carbenoid? *J. Am. Chem. Soc.* **2004**, *126*, 15795–15801. [CrossRef] [PubMed]
8. Vyanakaram, K.; Havlas, Z.; Michl, J. Aromatic substitution with *hypercloso* $C(BCH_3)_{11}$: A new mechanism. *J. Am. Chem. Soc.* **2007**, *129*, 4172–4174. [CrossRef] [PubMed]
9. Thomas, S.P.; Pavan, M.S.; Guru Row, T.N. Experimental evidence for 'carbon bonding' in the solid state from charge density analysis. *Chem. Commun.* **2014**, *50*, 49–51. [CrossRef]
10. Alkorta, I.; Rozas, I.; Elguero, J. Molecular complexes between silicon derivatives and electron-rich groups. *J. Phys. Chem. A* **2001**, *105*, 743–749. [CrossRef]
11. Bauzá, A.; Mooibroek, T.J.; Frontera, A. Tetrel-bonding interaction: Rediscovered supramolecular force? *Angew. Chem. Int. Ed.* **2013**, *52*, 12317–12321. [CrossRef] [PubMed]
12. Grabowski, S.J. Tetrel bond–σ-hole bond as a preliminary stage of the S_N2 reaction. *Phys. Chem. Chem. Phys.* **2014**, *16*, 1824–1834. [CrossRef]
13. Curtiss, L.A.; Redfern, P.C.; Raghavachari, K. Gaussian-4 theory using reduced order perturbation theory. *J. Chem. Phys.* **2007**, *127*, 124105. [CrossRef] [PubMed]
14. Frisch, M.J.; Trucks, G.W.; Schlegel, H.B.; Scuseria, G.E.; Robb, M.A.; Cheeseman, J.R.; Scalmani, G.; Barone, V.; Petersson, G.A.; Nakatsuji, H.; et al. *Gaussian 16; Revision C.01*; Gaussian Inc.: Wallingford, CT, USA, 2016.
15. Hohenberg, P.; Kohn, W. Inhomogeneous electron gas. *Phys. Rev.* **1964**, *136*, B864–B871. [CrossRef]
16. Kohn, W.; Sham, L.J. Self-consistent equations including exchange and correlation effects. *Phys. Rev.* **1965**, *140*, A1133–A1138. [CrossRef]
17. Møller, C.; Plesset, M.S. Note on an approximation treatment for many-electron systems. *Phys. Rev.* **1934**, *46*, 618–622. [CrossRef]
18. Bader, R.F.W. *Atoms in Molecules: A Quantum Theory*; Clarendon Press: Oxford, UK, 1990.
19. Popelier, P.L.A. *Atoms in Molecules. An Introduction*; Prentice Hall: Harlow, UK, 2000.

20. Keith, T.A. *AIMAll*; Version 19.10.12; TK Gristmill Software: Overland Park, KS, USA, 2017.
21. Silvi, B.; Savin, A. Classification of chemical bonds based on topological analysis of electron localization functions. *Nature* **1994**, *371*, 683–686. [CrossRef]
22. Becke, A.D.; Edgecombe, K.E. A simple measure of electron localization in atomic and molecular systems. *J. Chem. Phys.* **1990**, *92*, 5397–5403. [CrossRef]
23. Noury, S.; Krokidis, X.; Fuster, F.; Silvi, B. *TopMod Package*; Universite Pierre et Marie Curie: Paris, France, 1997.
24. Mata, I.; Alkorta, I.; Molins, E.; Espinosa, E. Universal features of the electron density distribution in hydrogen-bonding regions: A comprehensive study involving H···X (X=H, C, N, O, F, S, Cl, π) interactions. *Chem. Eur. J.* **2010**, *16*, 2442–2452. [CrossRef]
25. Alkorta, I.; Solimannejad, M.; Provasi, P.F.; Elguero, J. Theoretical study of complexes and fluoride cation transfer between N_2F^+ and electron donors. *J. Phys. Chem. A* **2007**, *111*, 7154–7161. [CrossRef] [PubMed]
26. Sánchez-Sanz, G.; Trujillo, C.; Alkorta, I.; Elguero, J. Intermolecular weak interactions in HTexH dimers (X=O, S, Se, Te): Hydrogen bonds, chalcogen-chalcogen contacts and chiral discrimination. *ChemPhysChem* **2012**, *13*, 496–503. [CrossRef] [PubMed]
27. Alkorta, I.; Mata, I.; Molins, E.; Espinosa, E. Charged versus neutral hydrogen-bonded complexes: Is there a difference in the nature of the hydrogen bonds? *Chem. Eur. J.* **2016**, *22*, 9226–9234. [CrossRef] [PubMed]
28. Savin, A.; Jepsen, O.; Flad, J.; Andersen, O.K.; Preuss, H.; Von Schnering, H.G. Electron localization in solid-state structures of the elements: The diamond structure. *Angew. Chem. Int. Ed.* **1992**, *31*, 187–188. [CrossRef]
29. Heisenberg, W. Mehrkörperproblem und Resonanz in der Quantenmechanik. *Zeit. Phys.* **1985**, *38*, 456–471. [CrossRef]
30. Dirac, P.A.M. On the theory of quantum mechanics. *Proc. R. Soc. London. Ser. A Math. Phys. Sci.* **1926**, *112*, 661–677. [CrossRef]
31. Dontha, R.; Zhu, T.-C.; Shen, Y.; Wörle, M.; Hong, X.; Duttwyler, S. A 3D Analogue of phenyllithium: Solution-phase, solid-state, and computational study of the lithiacarborane $[Li{-}CB_{11}H_{11}]$. *Angew. Chem. Int. Ed. Engl.* **2019**, *58*, 19007–19013. [CrossRef] [PubMed]
32. Groom, C.R.; Bruno, I.J.; Lightfoot, M.P.; Ward, S.C. The Cambridge structural database. *Acta Crystallogr. B Struct. Sci. Cryst. Eng. Mater.* **2016**, *B72*, 171–179. [CrossRef] [PubMed]
33. Pecyna, J.; Ringstrand, B.; Domagała, S.; Kaszyński, P.; Woźniak, K. Synthesis and characterization of 12-pyridinium derivatives of the [*closo*-1-$CB_{11}H_{12}]^-$ anion. *Inorg. Chem.* **2014**, *53*, 12617–12626. [CrossRef]
34. Douglass, A.G.; Janousek, Z.; Kaszynski, P.; Young, V.G., Jr. Synthesis and molecular structure of 12-iodo-1-(4-pentylquinuclidin-1-yl)-1-carba-*closo*-dodecaborane. *Inorg. Chem.* **1998**, *37*, 6361–6365. [CrossRef]
35. Finze, M.; Sprenger, J.A.P. 1-amino-2-fluoromonocarba-*closo*-dodecaborates: K[1-H_2N-2-F-*closo*-1-$CB_{11}H_{10}$] and [Et_4N][1-H_2N-2-F-*closo*-1-$CB_{11}I_{10}$]. *Z. Anorg. Allg. Chem.* **2010**, *636*, 1538–1542. [CrossRef]
36. Pecyna, J.; Kaszynski, P.; Ringstrand, B.; Pociecha, D.; Pakhomov, S.; Douglass, A.G.; Young, V.G., Jr. Synthesis and characterization of quinuclidinium derivatives of the [*closo*-1-$CB_{11}H_{12}$]− anion as potential polar components of liquid crystal materials. *Inorg. Chem.* **2016**, *55*, 4016–4025. [CrossRef]
37. Maly, K.; Subrtova, V.; Petricek, V. Structure of 1-trimethylamine-1-carba-closo-dodecaborane(11). *Acta Crystallogr. Sect. C Cryst. Struct. Commun.* **1987**, *C43*, 593–594. [CrossRef]
38. Hailmann, M.; Herkert, L.; Himmelspach, A.; Finze, M. Difunctionalized {*closo*-1-CB_{11}} clusters: 1- and 2-amino-12-ethynylcarba-closo-dodecaborates. *Chem. Eur. J.* **2013**, *19*, 15745–15758. [CrossRef] [PubMed]
39. Morris, J.H.; Peters, G.S.; Spicer, M.D. 1-Me_2NH-2-CH_2Cl-*closo*-l-$CB_{11}H_{10}$. An unusual product from the insertion reaction of Me_2NBCl_2 with Li_2[7-Me_3N-*nido*-7-$CB_{10}H_{10}$]. *J. Organomet. Chem.* **1995**, *494*, 195–198. [CrossRef]

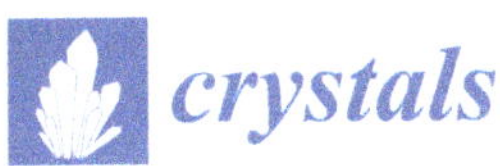
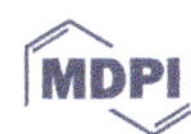

Article

Coordination Ability of 10-EtC(NHPr)=HN-7,8-$C_2B_9H_{11}$ in the Reactions with Nickel(II) Phosphine Complexes

Marina Yu. Stogniy [1,*], Svetlana A. Erokhina [1], Kyrill Yu. Suponitsky [1,2], Igor B. Sivaev [1] and Vladimir I. Bregadze [1]

1 A.N. Nesmeyanov Institute of Organoelement Compounds, Russian Academy of Science, 28 Vavilov Street, 119991 Moscow, Russia; hoborova.svetlana@yandex.ru (S.A.E.); kirshik@yahoo.com (K.Y.S.); sivaev@ineos.ac.ru (I.B.S.); bre@ineos.ac.ru (V.I.B.)
2 Basic Department of Chemistry of Innovative Materials and Technologies, G.V. Plekhanov Russian University of Economics, 36 Stremyannyi Line, 117997 Moscow, Russia
* Correspondence: stogniymarina@rambler.ru or stogniy@ineos.ac.ru

Abstract: The complexation reactions of *nido*-carboranyl amidine 10-PrNHC(Et)=HN-7,8-$C_2B_9H_{11}$ with different nickel(II) phosphine complexes such as [$(PR_2R')_2NiCl_2$] (R = R′ = Ph, Bu; R = Me, R′ = Ph) were investigated. As a result, a series of novel half-sandwich nickel(II) π,σ-complexes [3-R′R_2P-3-(8-Pr*N*=C(Et)NH)-*closo*-3,1,2-Ni$C_2B_9H_{10}$] with the coordination of the carborane and amidine components was prepared. The acidification of obtained complexes with HCl led to the breaking of the Ni-N bond with formation of nickel(II) π-complexes [3-Cl-3-R′R_2P-8-PrNH=C(Et)NH-*closo*-3,1,2-Ni$C_2B_9H_{10}$]. The crystal molecular structure of [3-Ph_3P-3-(8-Pr*N*=C(Et)NH)-*closo*-3,1,2-Ni$C_2B_9H_{10}$] was determined by single crystal X-ray diffraction.

Keywords: boron chemistry; *nido*-carborane; nitrilium derivatives; nickel(II) half sandwich complexes; synthesis; structure

Citation: Stogniy, M.Y.; Erokhina, S.A.; Suponitsky, K.Y.; Sivaev, I.B.; Bregadze, V.I. Coordination Ability of 10-EtC(NHPr)=HN-7,8-$C_2B_9H_{11}$ in the Reactions with Nickel(II) Phosphine Complexes. *Crystals* **2021**, *11*, 306. https://doi.org/10.3390/cryst11030306

Academic Editor: Alexander Kirillov

Received: 28 February 2021
Accepted: 16 March 2021
Published: 19 March 2021

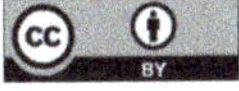

1. Introduction

The dicarbollide dianion $[7,8\text{-}C_2B_9H_{11}]^{2-}$, which is the deprotonated form of 7,8-dicarba-*nido*-undecaborate anion $[7,8\text{-}C_2B_9H_{12}]^-$ (*nido*-carborane), is known as the inorganic isolobal analogue of the cyclopentadienyl ligand. This makes it the perfect building block in complexation reactions with a wide range of transition metals [1–3]. The possibility to substitute hydrogen atoms at the carbon and boron vertices of the carborane cage with various functional groups [4] makes it possible to vary the properties of ligands based on *nido*-carborane by combining the properties of the *nido*-carborane nest with the properties of an exo-polyhedral substituent. One of the most interesting and promising tasks in this area is the synthesis of heterobifunctional *nido*-carborane-based ligands, that can give a firm bound to capture the metal center along with a weak bond, temporarily protecting a metal coordination site. This allows users to obtain labile complexes of transitional metal representing a promising new type of catalysts [5–10] and molecular switches [11,12]. There are several examples of such stable metal complexes based on *nido*-carborane with a side substituent coordinated through oxygen or nitrogen [5–8,13–15]. The utility of such bifunctional ligand systems with the nitrogen donor atom in the side chain has been demonstrated by the complexation of $[7\text{-}Me_2NCH_2\text{-}7,8\text{-}C_2B_9H_{11}]^-$ with metals such as nickel [16], iron [17], rhuthenium [17], titanium, zirconium, and hafnium [18,19]. In all cases, the intramolecular coordination of the dimethylamino group of the side substituent with the complexing metal was observed. The possibility of disrupting this coordination in the nickel(II) complexes by displacing the amino group with other soft ligands, such as triethylphosphine or *tert*-butylisocyanide, has been shown [16].

Earlier, we prepared a series of *nido*-carborane-based amidines 10-R$(CH_2)_n$NHC(Et)=HN-7,8-$C_2B_9H_{11}$ using the reaction of nucleophilic addition of amines to the 10-propionitrilium derivative of *nido*-carborane [20]. Therefore, it was of interest to study the possibility of using obtained amidines in the complexation reactions, where *nido*-carborane itself represents a firm π-acceptor and amidine nitrogen can act as an intramolecular protecting group. In this contribution we report synthesis of a series of new metallacarboranes by the reactions of *nido*-carborane-based amidine 10-PrNHC(Et)=HN-7,8-$C_2B_9H_{11}$ with nickel(II) phosphine complexes [$(R_2R'P)_2NiCl_2$].

2. Results and Discussion

Recently, we have shown the ease and simplicity of the modification of the *nido*-carborane moiety via nucleophilic addition reactions of various nucleophiles to the highly activated nitrilium group -N^+≡C-R attached to the cluster [20–22]. The nucleophilic addition of aliphatic and aromatic amines to the 10-propionitrilium derivative of *nido*-carborane (10-EtC≡N-7,8-$C_2B_9H_{11}$) leads to the formation of compounds that are a combination of the *nido*-carborane nest with the amidine fragment [20]. This promises the possibility of synthesizing complexes with simultaneous coordination of the carborane and amidine components. For our study we chose amidine 10-PrNHC(Et)=HN-7,8-$C_2B_9H_{11}$ (**1**) prepared by the nucleophilic addition of propyl amine to 10-EtC≡N-7,8-$C_2B_9H_{11}$. For the complexation reactions, we used nickel(II) phosphine complexes [$(R_2R'P)_2NiCl_2$] with ligands having different steric parameters (Tolman cone angles, θ)—$R_2R'P$ = Me_2PhP (θ = 122°), PBu_3 (θ = 132°), PPh_3 (θ = 145°) [23].

The addition of nickel(II) phosphine complexes [$(PR_2R')_2NiCl_2$] (R = R′ = Ph, Bu; R = Me, R′ = Ph) to a solution of the deprotonated amidine **1** in tetrahydrofuran at ambient temperature immediately led to a color change of the reaction mixtures color from pale yellow to dark red. Monitoring the progress of the reactions using thin layer chromatography showed that complexation occurs very quickly and is completed within 5-10 minutes. The column chromatography purification gave the corresponding π,σ-complexes [3-$R_2R'P$-3-(8-Pr*N*=C(Et)NH)-*closo*-3,1,2-$NiC_2B_9H_{10}$] (R = R′ = Ph (**2**), R = Me, R′ = Ph (**3**) and R = R′ = Bu (**4**)) in 80–83% yields (Scheme 1).

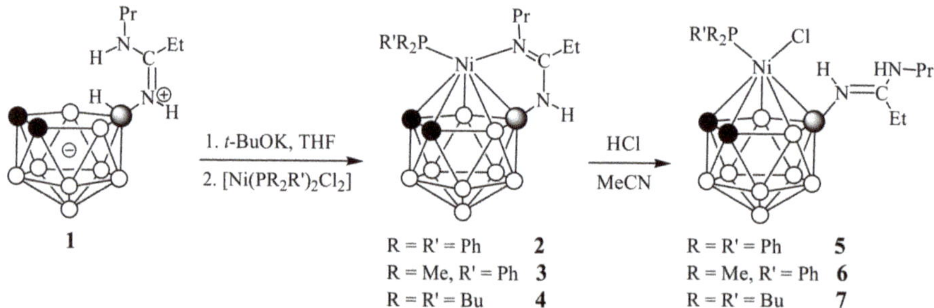

Scheme 1. Synthesis of nickelacarboranes **2–4** and **5–7**.

The initial analysis of the proposed structure of complexes **2–4** was carried out using standard methods of NMR and IR spectroscopy and mass spectrometry. The ^{1}H NMR spectra of complexes **2-4** demonstrated the presence of only one N*H* signal of the amidine substituent in the region of 5.04–5.53 ppm, as well as the absence of signals of the *nido*-carborane B-*H*-B bridge, suggesting that nickel was coordinated both by the pentagonal face of the carborane ligand and by one atom nitrogen of the amidine group. The pattern of the ^{11}B NMR spectra of complexes **2–4** is characteristic for metallacarboranes and consists of one singlet at ~4.0 ppm from the substituted boron atom and a set of four (complex **2**) or five (complexes **3** and **4**) doublets in the region from −11.2 to −27.4 ppm with total integral ratio of 1:2:3:2:1 (for **2**) and 1:2:2:1:2:1 (for **3** and **4**). The ^{1}H NMR spectra of complexes **2-4** also indicated the presence of a single phosphine ligand, while its ^{13}C NMR spectra demonstrated the characteristic splitting of signals from aromatic and/or aliphatic groups of phosphine ligands. In the ^{31}P NMR spectra, the signals of phosphine ligands appeared at 29.3 ppm for **2**, at −2.6 ppm for **3** and at 11.9 ppm for **4**. Such chemical shifts were in good agreement with the data for similar phosphine complexes of other transitional metals [24].

In the IR spectra of complexes **2–4**, the NH stretching bands were observed in the region of 3447–3244 cm^{-1}, whereas the BH stretching bands appeared at ~2530 cm^{-1}. The bands corresponding to the N=C bond were at ~1635 cm^{-1} for **2** and **3**, and at 1622 cm^{-1} for **4**. The mass spectra of complexes demonstrated only peak envelopes corresponding to molecular picks of the supposed structures of complexes **2–4**.

The suggested structures of complexes **2–4** were confirmed by single crystal X-ray diffraction study on complex **2** (Figure 1).

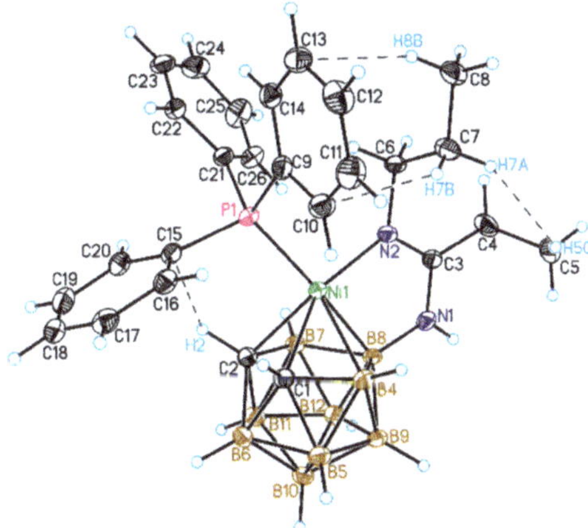

Figure 1. General view of the nickel(II) complex [3-Ph_3P-3-(8-Pr*N*=C(Et)NH)-*closo*-3,1,2-$NiC_2B_9H_{10}$] (**2**). Thermal ellipsoids are given at 50% probability level. Shortened contacts are shown by dashed lines.

The crystals of complex **2** suitable for X-ray analysis were obtained by slow evaporation from chloroform/hexane (3:1) solution. The nickel atom in the structure of **2** is approximately centered over the pentagonal face of the dicarbollide ligand with the Ni-C_2B_3 centroid distance of 1.526(2) Å. This is close to the distance found in a similar complex [3-Ph_3P-3-(8-$MeOCH_2CH_2$*N*=C(Et)NH)-3,1,2- $NiC_2B_9H_{10}$] (**2***) which differs only by a substituent at the N2 atom (1.533 Å) [25] and noticeably longer than in [3-Ph_3P-3-(1-Me_2NCH_2)-*closo*-3,1,2-$NiC_2B_9H_{10}$] (1.500 Å) [16], and shorter than in [3-Ph_3P-3-Cl-1-(*i*-PrNH)$_2$C-3,1,2-$NiC_2B_9H_{10}$] (1.564 Å) [26] and [3,3-$(Ph_3P)_2$-*closo*-3,1,2-$NiC_2B_9H_{11}$] (1.610 Å) [27]. The Ni-N and Ni-P bond lengths (1.914(2) and 2.2555(7) Å) are close to those found in **2*** (1.916 and 2.2532 Å) [25] and differ significantly from those found in [3-Ph_3P-3-(1-Me_2NCH_2)-*closo*-3,1,2-$NiC_2B_9H_{10}$] (2.061 and 2.166 Å, respectively) [16], reflecting the stronger electron-donating properties of the carboranylamidine ligand as compared to the carborane ligand with pendant NMe_2 group. A more detailed comparison of the structures of the complexes **2** and **2*** is presented in Table 1.

Table 1. Selected torsion angles (deg.), Ni-C_2B_3(centroid) distance and nonbonded intramolecular shortened contacts (Å) that define molecular conformation for experimental (X-ray) and calculated structure of complex **2** and comparison with **2***.

Structure Parameters	Compound 2 (X-ray)	Compound 2 *	Compound 2 (calc) *
Ni-C_2B_3(centroid)	1.526 (2)	1.533 (2)	1.545
C2-Ni1-P1-C9	143.7 (2)	128.3 (2)	125.5
C2-Ni1-P1-C15	26.3 (2)	8.3 (2)	8.0
C2-Ni1-P1-C21	−93.3 (2)	−108.9 (2)	−110.5
B8-N1-C3-C4	−179.0 (2)	−174.1 (2)	172.0
N1-C3-C4-C5	−63.2 (2)	100.0 (2)	−62.1
Ni1-N2-C6-C7	104.7 (2)	85.1 (2)	95.9
H2 … C15	2.66	2.54	2.45 (−2.5)
H7B … C10	2.76	2.75	2.74 (−1.1)
H8B … C13	3.04	-	2.98 (−0.7)
H5C … H7A	2.37	2.28 (H5C … H6B)	2.30 (−1.0)

* for noncovalent contacts, their attractive energies in kcal/mol are given in parenthesis.

The Ni-C_2B_3 centroid distances were only slightly different, and differences in orientation of the PPh_3 fragment were not so pronounced (within 15° of rotation about Ni-P bond). The most significant unequivalence, as expected, was observed for substituents at the N2 and C3 atoms. In spite of that, the system of shortened contacts was quite similar. One can suggest that the observed conformation can be stabilized by intramolecular noncovalent interactions. To confirm that, we carried out quantum chemical calculations of complex **2**. In optimized structure, torsion angles, which define the orientation of PPh_3 fragment, differ by ca. 18° while differences in orientation of the ethyl and propyl groups are less pronounced. Again, the system of shortened contacts, for which bond critical point were localized, was still nearly the same. Those contacts in total added −5.3 kcal/mol to the stabilization of molecular conformation. These results suggest that the variation of substituents at the N2 and C3 atoms would not significantly affect the orientation of the PPh_3 fragment relative to the carborane cage.

An attempt to obtain suitable X-ray diffraction study crystals of **3** and **4** by recrystallization from chloroform unexpectedly led to a change in the color of the solution from dark red to amaranth after ~12 h. Thin layer chromatography confirmed the formation of a new product together with the presence of small amounts of original complexes **3** and **4**. New complexes **6** and **7** were isolated by column chromatography on silica using dichloromethane as an eluent. An analysis of the NMR spectra of complexes **6** and **7** led to the assumption that the metal atom in the obtained complexes was no longer coordinated by the amidine group (Figure 2).

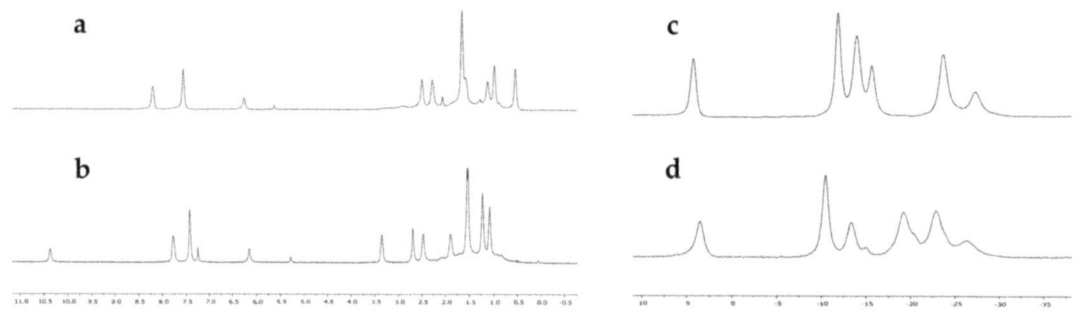

Figure 2. ^{1}H NMR spectra of complexes **3** (**a**) and **6** (**b**) and $^{11}B\{^{1}H\}$ NMR spectra of complexes **3** (**c**) and **6** (**d**).

In the ^{1}H NMR spectra of complexes **6** and **7**, signals from the second N*H* proton appeared in low field at 10.37 and 9.90 ppm for **6** and **7**, respectively (Figure 2, items a,b). This signal gave cross-pick in the ^{1}H-^{1}H COSY NMR spectrum with the methylene group of the propyl group -C*H*$_2$CH$_2$CH$_3$ (See SI). The ^{11}B NMR spectra of **6** and **7** confirmed the retention of the metallacarborane skeleton, however their spectral patterns differed from those for complexes **3** and **4** (Figure 2, items c,d). Since the newly formed complexes were neutral, we assumed that the violation of the coordination of the amidine fragment was caused by the protonation of the second nitrogen atom, and the electroneutrality of the complexes was achieved due to the coordination of the chloride ion by the nickel atom. The driving force behind this process could be the trace amounts of hydrogen chloride normally present in chloroform. To verify this assumption, we resynthesized complexes **3** and **4**, dissolved them in acetonitrile and acidified them by small amounts of concentrated hydrochloric acid (Scheme 1). This resulted in an immediate change in color of the complexes from dark red to amaranth (Figure 3). The NMR spectra confirmed the formation of complexes **6** and **7** (See SM).

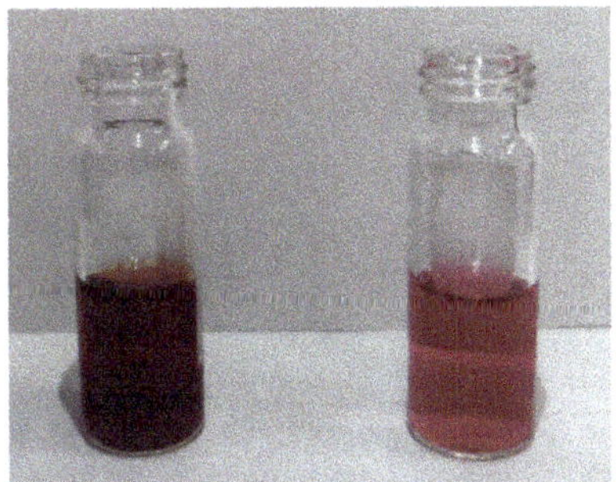

Figure 3. The color of complex **4** (left) and complex **7** (right).

For complex **2**, which did not change upon standing in chloroform solution, we carried out a similar acidification procedure with hydrochloric acid. The solution immediately changed its color from dark red to amaranth, but, unlike complexes **3** and **4**, the transformation of complex **2** into a similar complex **5** was not complete. According to the NMR spectroscopy data, the reaction mixture contained approximately 90% of complex **5** and ~10% of the original complex **2** and the addition of more amounts of hydrochloric acid did not change this ratio. An attempt to purify complex **5** by column chromatography on silica gel with dichloromethane as an eluent resulted in a mixture of complexes **2** and **5** with a new ratio of ~5:2, which can be caused by the presence of equilibrium between these complexes and the partial loss of chloride ions on the column (Scheme 2).

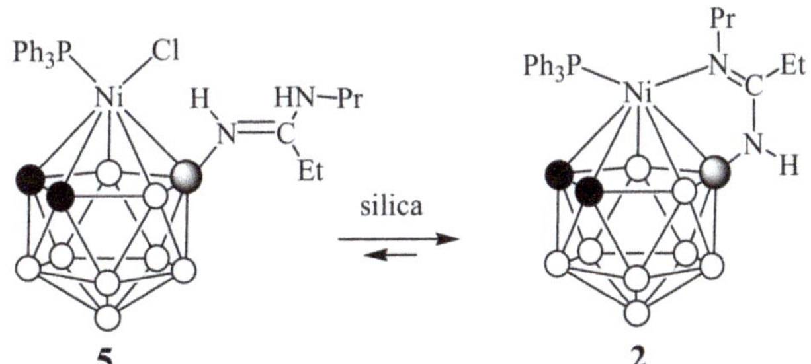

Scheme 2. Behavior of complex **5** during purification on column chromatography with silica gel.

We supposed that the less donor PPh_3 ligand made the Ni-N bond in complex **2** stronger than in complexes **3** and **4** with more donor phosphine ligands PMe_2Ph and PBu_3.

Like complexes **6** and **7**, the ^{1}H NMR spectrum of complex **5** contained the signals of two different *NH* protons: one at 9.09 ppm from the *NH*Pr group and another one at 5.53 ppm from the B-*NH*-C fragment. However, in contrast to complexes **2–4** in the ^{1}H NMR spectra of **5–7**, the signals of the CH_{carb} groups appeared in low-field at 2.57–2.80 ppm (0.44–1.12 ppm for complexes **2–4**). The signals of the ethyl and propyl group of the amidine substituent in **5–7** also underwent a number of changes and in general were shifted to the low field. For example, the signal of the methylene group of the propyl fragment -NHC***H***$_2$CH$_2$CH$_3$ in complex **7** was observed at 3.41 ppm, whereas in complex **4** it appeared at 2.75 ppm. The signal of the methylene group of the ethyl substituent was located at 2.54 ppm for **7** in contrast with 2.22 ppm for **4**. At the same time, the signals of the carbon atom of the methylene group of the propyl fragment -NHCH$_2$CH$_2$CH$_3$ in ^{13}C NMR spectra of **5–7** underwent the high field shift from ~55 ppm for **2–4** to ~46 ppm, whereas the signal of the methylene group of the ethyl fragment demonstrated a slight high field shift from ~23–24 ppm for **2–4** to ~26–30 ppm for **5–7**. In the ^{11}B NMR spectra of complexes **5–7**, the singlet from the substituted boron atom was observed at 1.9 ppm for **5** and at 3.5 ppm for **6** and **7**. Other signals appeared as groups of four (complex **5**) or five (complexes **6** and **7**) doublets in the region from -10.2 to -26.3 ppm with the total integral ratios 1:2:1:4:1 for **5** and 1:2:1:2:2:1 for **6** and **7**. The chemical shifts of phosphine ligands in the ^{31}P NMR spectra of **5–7** were close to those for **2–4**. In the IR spectra of **5–7**, the NH and BH stretching bands were observed in the region of 3402–3223 cm^{-1} and ~2555 cm^{-1}, respectively, whereas the bands corresponding to the N=C bond appeared at 1632, 1626 and 1630 cm^{-1} for **5**, **6** and **7**, respectively. The mass spectra of complexes **5–7** performed using the MS MALDI technique contained two main sets of signals corresponding to the molecular picks of complexes **5–7** themselves and complexed with the loss of the chloride ligand. For example, the MALDI mass spectrum of complex **6** contained a typical carborane envelope centered at m/z 477.253 corresponding to the molecular ion pick and another one centered at m/z 442.275, that corresponded to the loss of the chloride ligand by complex **6**.

3. Conclusions

In this work the utility of using the *nido*-carboranyl amidine 10-PrNHC(Et)=HN-7,8-$C_2B_9H_{11}$ in the complexation reactions with different nickel(II) phosphine complexes was demonstrated. As a result, a series of novel half-sandwich nickel(II) π,σ-complexes [3-R$_2$R′P-3-(8-Pr*N*=C(Et)NH)-*closo*-3,1,2-NiC$_2$B$_9$H$_{10}$] (R = R′ = Ph, Bu; R = Me, R′ = Ph) was prepared. The crystal molecular structure of [3-Ph$_3$P-3- (8-Pr*N*=C(Et)NH)-*closo*-3,1,2-NiC$_2$B$_9$H$_{10}$] was determined by single crystal X-ray diffraction. The acidification of obtained complexes with HCl led to the breaking of the Ni-N bond with the formation of the corresponding nickel(II) π-complexes [3-Cl-3-R′R$_2$P- 8-PrNH=C(Et)NH-*closo*-3,1,2-NiC$_2$B$_9$H$_{10}$] (R = R′ = Ph, Bu; R = Me, R′ = Ph). The process was accompanied by a change in the color of complexes from dark red to amaranth one. In this regard, the obtained complexes can be considered as potential acid-base indicators.

4. Experimental Section

4.1. Reagents and Methods

The amidine 10-PrNHC(Et)=HN-7,8-$C_2B_9H_{11}$ (**1**) was prepared according to procedure from the literature [20]. Dichlorobis(triphenylphosphine)nickel(II), dichlorobis (dimethylphenylphosphine)nickel(II) and dichlorobis(tributylphosphine)nickel(II) were synthesized according to the previously described methods [28]. Tetrahydrofuran was dried using standard procedure [29]. All manipulations were carried out in air. The reaction progress was monitored by thin-layer chromatography (Merck F254 silica gel on aluminum plates) and visualized using 0.5% $PdCl_2$ in 1% HCl in aq. MeOH (1:10). Acros Organics silica gel (0.060–0.200 mm) was used for column chromatography. The NMR spectra at 400.1 MHz (^{1}H), 128.4 MHz (^{11}B), 100.0 MHz (^{13}C) and 162 MHz (^{31}P) were recorded with a Varian Inova 400 spectrometer. The residual signal of the NMR solvent relative to tetramethylsilane was taken as an internal reference for ^{1}H and ^{13}C NMR spectra. ^{11}B NMR spectra were referenced using $BF_3 \cdot Et_2O$ as an external standard. ^{31}P NMR spectra were cited relative to 85% H_3PO_4 as an external standard. Infrared spectra were recorded on an IR Prestige-21 (SHIMADZU, Kyoto, Japan) instrument. UV/Vis spectra in chloroform were recorded with a SF-2000 spectrophotometer (OKB SPECTR LLC, Saint-Petersburg, Russia) using 1 cm cuvettes. MALDI mass spectra (positive ion mode) were acquired using a Bruker AutoFlex II reflector time-of-flight device equipped with an N_2 laser (337 nm, 2.5 ns pulse). *Trans*-2-[3-(4-*tert*-butylphenyl)-2-methyl-2-propenylidene]malononitrile (DCTB, ≥98%, Sigma-Aldrich, Louis, MO, USA) was chosen as a matrix, matrix-to-analyte molar ratio in spotted probes being more than 1000/1. High resolution mass spectra (HRMS) were measured on a Bruker micrOTOF II instrument using electrospray ionization (ESI). The measurements were done in a positive ion mode with mass range from m/z 50 to m/z 3000.

4.2. Synthesis of [3-Ph_3P-3-(8-PrN=C(Et)NH)-closo-3,1,2-$NiC_2B_9H_{10}$] (**2**)

The potassium *tert*-butoxide (0.34 g, 3.00 mmol) was added to a solution of **1** (0.15 g, 0.60 mmol) in dry tetrahydrofuran (15 mL). The mixture was stirred for ~10 min at room temperature and [$Ni(PPh_3)_2Cl_2$] (0.47 g, 0.72 mmol) was added by one portion. The pale-yellow color of the reaction mixture was immediately turned to dark red. The reaction mixture was stirred at room temperature in air for about 30 min and the solvent was evaporated under reduced pressure. The residue was treated with CH_2Cl_2 (20 mL) and water (20 mL). The insoluble particles were filtered off and the organic layer was separated, washed with water (2 × 20 mL) and evaporated under reduced pressure. The column chromatography on silica gel was used for the purification of the substance with hexane:CH_2Cl_2 (2:1) as an eluent to give maroon solid of **2** (0.28 g, 83% yield). The crystals suitable for X-ray analysis were obtained by slow evaporation from chloroform/hexane (3:1) solution.

^{1}H NMR ($CDCl_3$, ppm): δ 7.82 (6H, Ph), 7.44 (9H, Ph), 5.09 (1H, N*H*), 2.27 (2H, $NHCH_2CH_2CH_3$), 2.14 (2H, CH_2CH_3), 1.25 (2H, $NHCH_2CH_2CH_3$), 1.09 (3H, CH_2CH_3), 0.44 (2H, s, CH_{carb}), 0.04 (3H, $NHCH_2CH_2CH_3$), 3.4–0.2 (8H, br s, B*H*). ^{13}C NMR ($CDCl_3$, ppm): δ 176.9 (NH=C), 134.0 (*o*-Ph, d, J = 12 Hz), 131.2 (Ph, d, J = 37 Hz), 130.8 (*p*-Ph), 128.9 (*m*-Ph, d, J = 9 Hz), 56.1 ($NHCH_2CH_2CH_3$), 25.1 ($NHCH_2CH_2CH_3$), 24.0 (CH_2), 17.2 (CH_{carb}), 11.9 (CH_3), 10.4 ($NHCH_2CH_2CH_3$). ^{31}P NMR ($CDCl_3$, ppm): 29.3 (s, PPh_3). ^{11}B NMR ($CDCl_3$, ppm): δ 4.0 (1B, s), −11.2 (2B, d), −13.6 (3B, d), −23.5 (2B, d), −26.7 (1B, d). IR (film, cm^{-1}): 3437 ($\nu_{N\text{-}H}$), 3411 ($\nu_{N\text{-}H}$), 3308, 3245, 3057, 2966 ($\nu_{C\text{-}H}$), 2933 ($\nu_{C\text{-}H}$), 2875 ($\nu_{C\text{-}H}$), 2551 (br, $\nu_{B\text{-}H}$), 1635 ($\nu_{N=C}$), 1557, 1503, 1480, 1436, 1380, 1325, 1310. UV/VIS (λ, nm): 248, 330, 510. MALDI MS: m/z for $C_{26}H_{38}B_9N_2NiP$: calcd 565.299 $[M]^+$, obsd 565.288 $[M]^+$ (100).

4.3. Synthesis of [3-$PhMe_2P$-3-(8-PrN=C(Et)NH)-closo-3,1,2-$NiC_2B_9H_{10}$] (**3**)

The procedure was analogous to the preparation of **2** using **1** (0.13 g, 0.52 mmol), potassium *tert*-butoxide (0.30 g, 2.60 mmol) and [$Ni(PMe_2Ph)_2Cl_2$] (0.25 g, 0.62 mmol) in dry tetrahydrofuran (15 mL). The column chromatography on silica gel was used for the purification of the substance with CH_2Cl_2 as an eluent to give maroon solid of **3** (0.19 g, 82% yield).

^{1}H NMR (acetone-d_6, ppm): δ 8.19 (2H, Ph), 7.54 (3H, Ph), 6.25 (1H, N*H*), 2.48 (2H, $NHCH_2CH_2CH_3$), 2.26 (2H, CH_2CH_3), 1.65 (6H, $P(CH_3)_2$), 1.57 (2H, $NHCH_2CH_2CH_3$), 1.12 (2H, s, CH_{carb}), 0.98 (3H, CH_2CH_3), 0.53 (3H, $NHCH_2CH_2CH_3$), 3.4–0.4 (8H, br s, B*H*). ^{13}C NMR (acetone-d_6, ppm): δ 177.7 (NH=C), 131.3 (Ph, d, J = 18 Hz), 131.2 (*o*-Ph, d, J = 12 Hz), 130.3 (*p*-Ph), 128.8 (*m*-Ph, d, J = 10 Hz), 54.3 ($NHCH_2CH_2CH_3$), 26.5 ($NHCH_2CH_2CH_3$), 23.4 (CH_2), 14.7 (CH_{carb}), 13.7 ($P(CH_3)_2$, d, J = 24 Hz), 11.7 (CH_3), 10.3 ($NHCH_2CH_2CH_3$). ^{31}P NMR (acetone-d_6, ppm): −2.6 (s, PMe_2Ph). ^{11}B NMR (acetone-d_6, ppm): δ 4.2 (1B, s), −12.0 (2B, d, J = 137 Hz), −14.0 (2B, d, J = 156 Hz), −15.7 (1B, d, J = 147 Hz), −23.8 (2B, d, J = 143 Hz), −27.4 (1B, d, J = 144 Hz). IR (film, cm^{-1}): 3410 ($\nu_{N\text{-}H}$), 3244 ($\nu_{N\text{-}H}$), 2962

($\nu_{C\text{-}H}$), 2930 ($\nu_{C\text{-}H}$), 2874 ($\nu_{C\text{-}H}$), 2525 (br, $\nu_{B\text{-}H}$), 1636 ($\nu_{N=C}$), 1568, 1493, 1437, 1377, 1300, 1292. ESI HRMS: *m/z* for $C_{16}H_{34}B_9N_2NiP$: calcd 441.2696 $[M]^+$, obsd 441.2696 $[M]^+$ (100).

4.4. Synthesis of [3-Bu_3P-3-(8-PrN=C(Et)NH)-closo-3,1,2-$NiC_2B_9H_{10}$] (**4**)

The procedure was analogous to the preparation of **2** using **1** (0.16 g, 0.64 mmol), potassium *tert*-butoxide (0.36 g, 3.20 mmol) and $[Ni(PBu_3)_2Cl_2]$ (0.26 g, 0.77 mmol) in dry tetrahydrofuran (15 mL). The column chromatography on silica gel was used for the purification of the substance with CH_2Cl_2 as an eluent to give maroon solid of **3** (0.25 g, 80% yield).

^{1}H NMR ($CDCl_3$, ppm): δ 5.04 (1H, N*H*), 2.75 (2H, $NHCH_2CH_2CH_3$), 2.22 (2H, CH_2CH_3), 1.70 (2H, $NHCH_2CH_2CH_3$), 1.61 (6H, $P(CH_2CH_2CH_2CH_3)_3$), 1.50 (6H, $P(CH_2CH_2CH_2CH_3)_3$), 1.40 (6H, $P(CH_2CH_2CH_2CH_3)_3$), 1.06 (3H, CH_2CH_3), 0.93 (14H, $NHCH_2CH_2CH_3$ + $P(CH_2CH_2CH_2CH_3)_3$ + CH_{carb}), 3.4–0.2 (8H, br s, B*H*). ^{13}C NMR ($CDCl_3$, ppm): δ 176.6 (NH=C), 55.2 ($NHCH_2CH_2CH_3$), 26.7 ($NHCH_2CH_2CH_3$), 26.5 ($P(CH_2CH_2CH_2CH_3)_3$, d, J = 50 Hz), 24.4 ($P(CH_2CH_2CH_2CH_3)_3$, d, J = 12 Hz), 24.2 (CH_2), 23.5 ($P(CH_2CH_2CH_2CH_3)_3$, d, J = 20 Hz), 14.0 (CH_{carb}), 13.7 ($P(CH_2CH_2CH_2CH_3)_3$), 11.8 (CH_3), 11.5 ($NHCH_2CH_2CH_3$). ^{31}P NMR ($CDCl_3$, ppm): 11.9 (s, PBu_3). ^{11}B NMR ($CDCl_3$, ppm): δ 3.8 (1B, s), −11.8 (2B, d), −14.3 (2B, d), −15.1 (1B, d), −23.6 (2B, d), −26.8 (1B, d). IR (film, cm^{-1}): 3447 ($\nu_{N\text{-}H}$), 3408 ($\nu_{N\text{-}H}$), 2957 ($\nu_{C\text{-}H}$), 2932 ($\nu_{C\text{-}H}$), 2872 ($\nu_{C\text{-}H}$), 2544 (br, $\nu_{B\text{-}H}$), 1622 ($\nu_{N=C}$), 1557, 1497, 1464, 1379, 1283. MALDI MS: *m/z* for $C_{20}H_{50}B_9N_2NiP$: calcd 506.402 $[M+H]^+$, obsd 506.400 $[M+H]^+$ (100).

4.5. General Procedure for the Synthesis of [3-Cl-3-$R'R_2P$-8-PrN=C(Et)NH-closo-3,1,2-$NiC_2B_9H_{10}$] (**5–7**)

To the *N*-coordinated complexes **2–4** (0.40 mmol) dissolved in MeCN (10 mL), one drop (~0.1 mL) of concentrated HCl was added at room temperature. The dark red color of solution was immediately changed to amaranth. The solution was stirred for 5 min and evaporated under reduced pressure to give amaranth solid of **5–7.** In the case of complexes **6** and **7**, the column chromatography on silica gel was used for the purification with CH_2Cl_2 as an eluent.

Spectral data for [3-Cl-3-Ph_3P-8-Pr*N*=C(Et)NH-*closo*-3,1,2-$NiC_2B_9H_{10}$] (**5**)

Yield 0.18 g (75%).

^{1}H NMR ($CDCl_3$, ppm): δ 9.09 (1H, N*H*Pr), 7.62 (6H, Ph), 7.31 (9H, Ph), 5.53 (1H, N*H*), 3.22 (2H, $NHCH_2CH_2CH_3$), 2.57 (2H, CH_{carb}), 1.86 (4H, $NHCH_2CH_2CH_3$ + CH_2CH_3), 0.93 (6H, $NHCH_2CH_2CH_3$ + CH_2CH_3), 3.8–0.3 (8H, br s, B*H*). ^{13}C NMR ($CDCl_3$, ppm): δ 167.5 (NH=C), 134.3 (Ph), 133.7 (Ph), 130.4 (Ph), 128.2 (Ph), 45.6 ($NHCH_2CH_2CH_3$), 30.8 (CH_2), 25.2 ($NHCH_2CH_2CH_3$), 23.2 (CH_{carb}), 11.1 (CH_3), 9.8 ($NHCH_2CH_2CH_3$). ^{31}P NMR ($CDCl_3$, ppm): 28.2 (s, PPh_3). ^{11}B NMR ($CDCl_3$, ppm): δ 1.9 (1B, s), −10.2 (2B, d), −12.3 (1B, d), −20.8 (4B, d), −24.2 (1B, d). IR (film, cm^{-1}): 3397 ($\nu_{N\text{-}H}$), 3302 ($\nu_{N\text{-}H}$), 3233 ($\nu_{N\text{-}H}$), 3059, 2966 ($\nu_{C\text{-}H}$), 2967 ($\nu_{C\text{-}H}$), 2928 ($\nu_{C\text{-}H}$), 2878 ($\nu_{C\text{-}H}$), 2560 (br, $\nu_{B\text{-}H}$), 1632 ($\nu_{N=C}$), 1553, 1501, 1481, 1437, 1385, 1259. UV/VIS (λ, nm): 280, 302, 486. MALDI MS: *m/z* for $C_{26}H_{39}B_9N_2ClNiP$: calcd 601.277 $[M]^+$, obsd 601.293 $[M]^+$ (10), *m/z* for $C_{26}H_{39}B_9N_2NiP$: calcd 566.308 $[M\text{-}Cl]^+$, obsd 566.321 $[M\text{-}Cl]^+$ (90).

Spectral data for [3-Cl-3-$PhMe_2P$-8-Pr*N*=C(Et)NH-*closo*-3,1,2-$NiC_2B_9H_{10}$] (**6**)

Yield 0.16 g (84%).

^{1}H NMR (acetone-d_6, ppm): δ 10.37 (1H, N*H*Pr), 7.77 (2H, Ph), 7.42 (3H, Ph), 6.15 (1H, N*H*), 3.35 (2H, $NHCH_2CH_2CH_3$), 2.69 (2H, s, CH_{carb}), 2.48 (2H, CH_2CH_3), 1.89 (2H, $NHCH_2CH_2CH_3$), 1.53 (6H, $P(CH_3)_2$), 1.23 (3H, CH_2CH_3), 1.08 (3H, $NHCH_2CH_2CH_3$), 3.0–0.5 (8H, br s, B*H*). ^{13}C NMR (acetone-d_6, ppm): δ 130.2 (Ph), 130.0 (Ph), 129.0 (Ph), 46.1 ($NHCH_2CH_2CH_3$), 26.2 (CH_2), 23.4 ($NHCH_2CH_2CH_3$), 14.8 ($P(CH_3)_2$), 11.7 ($NHCH_2CH_2CH_3$), 9.7 (CH_3). ^{31}P NMR (acetone-d_6, ppm): −2.53 (s, PMe_2Ph). ^{11}B NMR (acetone-d_6, ppm): δ 3.5 (1B, s), −10.5 (2B, d, J = 133 Hz), −13.4 (1B, d, J = 145 Hz), −19.2 (2B, d, J = 140 Hz), −22.9 (2B, d, J = 117 Hz), −26.3 (1B, d, J = 172 Hz). IR (film, cm^{-1}): 3402 ($\nu_{N\text{-}H}$), 3259 ($\nu_{N\text{-}H}$), 3227 ($\nu_{N\text{-}H}$), 3053, 2968 ($\nu_{C\text{-}H}$), 2934 ($\nu_{C\text{-}H}$), 2878 ($\nu_{C\text{-}H}$), 2548 (br, $\nu_{B\text{-}H}$), 1626 ($\nu_{N=C}$), 1557, 1435, 1421, 1384, 1361, 1296. MALDI MS: *m/z* for $C_{16}H_{35}B_9N_2ClNiP$: calcd 477.245

$[M]^+$, obsd 477.253 $[M]^+$ (23), m/z for $C_{16}H_{35}B_9N_2NiP$: calcd 442.276 $[M-Cl]^+$, obsd 442.275 $[M-Cl]^+$ (77).

Spectral data for [3-Cl-3-Bu_3P-8-Pr*N*=C(Et)NH-*closo*-3,1,2-$NiC_2B_9H_{10}$] (**7**)

Yield 0.19 g (88%).

^1H NMR ($CDCl_3$, ppm): δ 9.90 (1H, N*H*Pr), 6.22 (1H, N*H*), 3.41 (2H, q, J = 7.5 Hz, $NHCH_2CH_2CH_3$), 2.80 (2H, s, CH_{carb}), 2.54 (2H, q, J = 7.6 Hz, CH_2CH_3), 1.90 (2H, m, J = 7.5 Hz, $NHCH_2CH_2CH_3$), 1.58 (12H, $P(CH_2CH_2CH_2CH_3)_3$), 1.39 (6H, $P(CH_2CH_2CH_2CH_3)_3$), 1.28 (3H, t, J = 7.6 Hz, CH_2CH_3), 1.07 (3H, t, J = 7.5 Hz, $NHCH_2CH_2CH_3$), 0.93 (9H, $P(CH_2CH_2CH_2CH_3)_3$), 3.3–0.9 (8H, br s, B*H*). ^{13}C NMR ($CDCl_3$, ppm): δ 46.2 ($NHCH_2CH_2CH_3$), 30.8 (CH_{carb}), 26.3 (CH_2), 26.2 ($P(CH_2CH_2CH_2CH_3)_3$), 24.5 ($P(CH_2CH_2CH_2CH_3)_3$), 23.7 ($P(CH_2CH_2CH_2CH_3)_3$, 23.6 ($NHCH_2CH_2CH_3$), 11.6 ($NHCH_2CH_2CH_3$), 10.3 (CH_3), 13.8 ($P(CH_2CH_2CH_2CH_3)_3$). ^{31}P NMR ($CDCl_3$, ppm): 11.7 (s, PBu_3). ^{11}B NMR ($CDCl_3$, ppm): δ 3.5 (1B, s), −10.6 (2B, d, J = 127 Hz), −13.9 (1B, d, J = 129 Hz), −20.3 (2B, d, J = 135 Hz), −23.7 (2B, d), −26.3 (1B, d). IR (film, cm^{-1}): 3223 ($\nu_{N\text{-}H}$), 2957 ($\nu_{C\text{-}H}$), 2930 ($\nu_{C\text{-}H}$), 2872 ($\nu_{C\text{-}H}$), 2550 (br, $\nu_{B\text{-}H}$), 1630 ($\nu_{N=C}$), 1552, 1462, 1415, 1379, 1342, 1300. UV/VIS (λ, nm): 246, 324, 517. MALDI MS: m/z for $C_{20}H_{51}B_9N_2ClNiP$: calcd 541.371 $[M]^+$, obsd 541.373 $[M]^+$ (9) m/z for $C_{20}H_{51}B_9N_2NiP$: calcd 506.402 $[M-Cl]^+$, obsd 506.443 $[M-Cl]^+$ (91).

4.6. Single Crystal X-ray Diffraction Study

X-ray experiment for compound **2** was carried out using a SMART APEX2 CCD diffractometer (λ(Mo-Kα) = 0.71073 Å, graphite monochromator, ω-scans) at 120 K. Collected data were processed by the SAINT and SADABS programs incorporated into the APEX2 program package [30]. The structure was solved by direct methods and refined by the full-matrix least-squares procedure against F^2 in anisotropic approximation. The refinement was carried out with the SHELXTL program [31]. The CCDC number 2065468 contains the supplementary crystallographic data (Supplementary Materials) for this paper. These data can be obtained free of charge via www.ccdc.cam.ac.uk/data_request/cif (accessed on 19 March 2021).

Crystallographic data for **2**: $C_{26}H_{38}B_9NiN_2P \cdot CHCl_3$ are triclinic, space group *P*-1: a = 10.0074(6) Å, b = 11.0974(6) Å, c = 16.8683(8) Å, α = 76.8900(10)°, β = 81.3380(10)°, γ = 67.4720(10)°, V = 1681.05(16) Å^3, Z = 2, M = 684.92, d_{cryst} = 1.353 g·cm^{-3}. $wR2$= 0.1312 calculated on F^2_{hkl} for all 8953 independent reflections with $2\theta < 58.3°$, (GOF = 1.048, R = 0.0528 calculated on F_{hkl} for 6268 reflections with $I > 2\sigma(I)$).

4.7. Quantum Chemical Calculation

Optimization of the geometry of compound **2** was carried out using the Gaussian program [32] at PBE0/def2tzvp level of approximation, which was adopted in our earlier calculations [33–36]. The AIM theory [37,38] was utilized to search for bond critical points of molecular electron density. Correlation of interatomic energy and potential energy density at bond critical point (E=1/2V(r)) [39,40] was adopted for estimation of the energy of noncovalent intramolecular interactions taking into account its reliability for energetic analysis [41–43].

Supplementary Materials: The following are available online at https://www.mdpi.com/2073-4352/11/3/306/s1. Figure S1–S29 NMR spectra of compounds **2**–**7**.

Author Contributions: Synthesis and writing, NMR, IR research analysis, M.Y.S.; synthesis, S.A.E.; X-ray diffraction study, K.Y.S.; supervision, writing, I.B.S.; editing V.I.B. All authors have read and agreed to the published version of the manuscript.

Funding: This work was supported by the Russian Science Foundation (№ 19-73-00229).

Institutional Review Board Statement: Not applicable.

Informed Consent Statement: Not applicable.

Data Availability Statement: The data presented in this study are available in Supplementary Materials.

Acknowledgments: The NMR spectroscopy and X-ray diffraction experiments were performed using equipment of the Center for Molecular Structure Studies at A.N. Nesmeyanov Institute of Organoelement Compounds, operating with financial support of the Ministry of Science and Higher Education of the Russian Federation. The authors thank Vitaliy Yu. Markov (M.V. Lomonosov Moscow State University) for collecting MALDI mass spectra.

Conflicts of Interest: The authors declare no conflict of interest.

References

1. Grimes, R.N. Transitional metal metallacarbaboranes. In *Comprehensive Organometallic Chemistry II*; Elsevier: Oxford, UK, 1995; Volume 1, pp. 373–430.
2. Grimes, R.N. Metallacarboranes in the new millennium. *Coord. Chem. Rev.* **2000**, *200*, 773–811. [CrossRef]
3. Hosmane, N.S.; Maguire, J.A. Metallacarboranes of *d*- and *f*-block metals. In *Comprehensive Organometallic Chemistry III*; Elsevier: Oxford, UK, 2007; Volume 3, pp. 175–264.
4. Bregadze, V.I. Dicarba-*closo*-dodecaboranes $C_2B_{10}H_{12}$ and their derivatives. *Chem. Rev.* **1992**, *92*, 209–223. [CrossRef]
5. Yinghuai, Z.; Yulin, Z.; Carpenter, K.; Maguire, J.A.; Hosmane, N.S. Synthesis and catalytic activities of Group 4 metal complexes derived from $C_{(cage)}$-appended cyclohexyloxocarborane trianion. *J. Organomet. Chem.* **2005**, *690*, 2802–2808. [CrossRef]
6. Yinghuai, Z.; Lo Pei Sia, S.; Kooli, F.; Carpenter, K.; Kemp, R.A. Another example of carborane based trianionic ligand: Syntheses and catalytic activities of cyclohexylamino tailed ortho-carboranyl zirconium and titanium dicarbollides. *J. Organomet. Chem.* **2005**, *690*, 6284–6291. [CrossRef]
7. Shen, H.; Chan, H.-S.; Xie, Z. Guanylation of amines catalyzed by a half-sandwich titanacarborane amide complex. *Organometallics* **2006**, *25*, 5515–5517. [CrossRef]
8. Gao, M.; Tang, Y.; Xie, M.; Qian, C.; Xie, Z. Synthesis, structure, and olefin polymerization behavior of constrained-geometry Group 4 metallacarboranes incorporating imido-dicarbollyl ligands. *Organometallics* **2006**, *25*, 2578–2584. [CrossRef]
9. Shen, H.; Xie, Z. Titanacarborane Amide catalyzed transamination of guanidines. *Organometallics* **2008**, *27*, 2685–2687. [CrossRef]
10. Yinghuai, Z.; Hosmane, N.S. Carborane-based transitional metal complexes and their catalytic application for olefin polymerization: Current and future perspectives. *J. Organomet. Chem.* **2013**, *747*, 25–29. [CrossRef]
11. Sivaev, I.B. Ferrocene and transition metal bis(dicarbollides) as platform for design of rotatory molecular switches. *Molecules* **2017**, *22*, 2201. [CrossRef]
12. Anufriev, S.A.; Timofeev, S.V.; Anisimov, A.A.; Suponitsky, K.Y.; Sivaev, I.B. bis(dicarbollide) complexes of transition metals as a platform for molecular switches. Study of complexation of 8,8'-bis(methylsulfanyl) derivatives of cobalt and iron bis(dicarbollides). *Molecules* **2020**, *25*, 5745. [CrossRef] [PubMed]
13. Shen, H.; Chan, H.-S.; Xie, Z. Synthesis, structure, and reactivity of $[\sigma{:}\eta^1{:}\eta^5\text{-}(OCH_2)(Me_2NCH_2)C_2B_9H_9]Ti(NR_2)$ (R = Me, Et). *Organometallics* **2007**, *26*, 2694–2704. [CrossRef]
14. Lee, J.-D.; Lee, Y.-J.; Son, K.-C.; Han, W.-S.; Cheong, M.; Ko, J.; Kang, S.O. Synthesis, characterization, and reactivity of new types of constrained geometry Group 4 metal complexes derived from picolyl-substituted dicarbollide ligand systems. *J. Organomet. Chem.* **2007**, *692*, 5403–5413. [CrossRef]
15. Anufriev, S.A.; Sivaev, I.B.; Nakamura, H. Two possible ways to combine boron and gadolinium for Gd-quided BNCT. A concept. *Phosphorus Sulfur Silicon Relat. Elem.* **2020**, *195*, 910–917. [CrossRef]
16. Park, J.-S.; Kim, D.-H.; Kim, S.-J.; Ko, J.; Kim, S.H.; Cho, S.; Lee, C.-H.; Kang, S.O. Preparation and reactions of a half-sandwich dicarbollyl nickel(II) complexes containing a dimethylamino pendent group. *Organometallics* **2001**, *20*, 4483–4491. [CrossRef]
17. Park, J.-S.; Kim, D.-H.; Ko, J.; Kim, S.H.; Cho, S.; Lee, C.-H.; Kang, S.O. Half-sandwich iron(II) and ruthenium(II) complexes with the dicarbollylamino ligand system. *Organometallics* **2001**, *20*, 4632–4640. [CrossRef]
18. Kim, D.-H.; Won, J.H.; Kim, S.-J.; Ko, J.; Kim, S.H.; Cho, S.; Kang, S.O. Dicarbollide analogues of the constrained-geometry polymerization catalyst. *Organometallics* **2001**, *20*, 4298–4300. [CrossRef]
19. Lee, J.-D.; Lee, Y.-J.; Son, K.-C.; Cheong, M.; Ko, J.; Kang, S.O. New types of constrained geometry Group 4 metal complexes derived from the aminomethyldicarbollyl ligand system: Synthesis and structural characterization of mono-dicarbollylamino and bis-dicarbollylamino Group 4 metal complexes. *Organometallics* **2007**, *26*, 3374–3384. [CrossRef]
20. Stogniy, M.Y.; Erokhina, S.A.; Suponitsky, K.Y.; Anisimov, A.A.; Godovikov, I.A.; Sivaev, I.B.; Bregadze, V.I. Synthesis of novel carboranyl amidines. *J. Organomet. Chem.* **2020**, *909*, 121111. [CrossRef]
21. Stogniy, M.Y.; Erokhina, S.A.; Suponitsky, K.Y.; Anisimov, A.A.; Sivaev, I.B.; Bregadze, V.I. Nucleophilic addition reactions to the ethylnitrilium derivative of *nido*-carborane $10\text{-}EtC{\equiv}N\text{-}7,8\text{-}C_2B_9H_{11}$. *New J. Chem.* **2018**, *42*, 17958–17967. [CrossRef]
22. Stogniy, M.Y.; Erokhina, S.A.; Anisimov, A.A.; Suponitsky, K.Y.; Sivaev, I.B.; Bregadze, V.I. $10\text{-}NCCH_2CH_2OCH_2CH_2C{\equiv}N\text{-}7,8\text{-}C_2B_9H_{11}$: Synthesis and reactions with various nucleophiles. *Polyhedron* **2019**, *174*, 114170. [CrossRef]
23. Clavier, H.; Nolan, S.P. Percent buried volume for phosphine and *N*-heterocyclic carbene ligands: Steric properties in organometallic chemistry. *Chem. Commun.* **2010**, *46*, 841–861. [CrossRef]
24. Hunter, A.D.; Williams, T.R.; Zarzyczny, B.M.; Bottesch, H.W.; Dolan, S.A.; McDowell, K.A.; Thomas, D.N.; Mahler, C.H. Correlations among ^{31}P NMR coordination chemical shifts, Ru–P bond distances, and enthalpies of reaction in $Cp'Ru(PR_3)_2Cl$ complexes ($Cp' = \eta^5\text{-}C_5H_5, \eta^5\text{-}C_5Me_5$; $PR_3 = PMe_3, PPhMe_2, PPh_2Me, PPh_3, PEt_3, P^nBu_3$). *Organometallics* **2016**, *35*, 2701–2706. [CrossRef]

25. Stogniy, M.Y.; Erokhina, S.A.; Suponitsky, K.Y.; Markov, V.Y.; Sivaev, I.B. Synthesis and crystal structures of nickel(II) and palladium(II) complexes with *o*-carboranyl amidine ligands. *Dalton Trans.* **2021**, *50*. [CrossRef]
26. Yao, Z.-J.; Jin, G.-X. Synthesis, reactivity, and structural transformation of mono- and binuclear carboranylamidinate-based 3d metal complexes and metallacarborane derivatives. *Organometallics* **2012**, *31*, 1767–1774. [CrossRef]
27. Erdman, A.A.; Zubreichuk, Z.P.; Knizhnikov, V.A.; Maier, A.A.; Aleksandrov, G.G.; Nefedov, S.E.; Eremenko, I.L. Synthesis and the structure of the triphenylphosphine complex of *o*-nickelacarborane, 3,3-$(PPh_3)_2$-3,1,2-$NiC_2B_9H_{11}$. *Russ. Chem. Bull.* **2001**, *50*, 2248–2250. [CrossRef]
28. Standley, E.A.; Smith, S.J.; Müller, P.; Jamison, T.F. A broadly applicable strategy for entry into homogeneous nickel(0) catalysts from air-stable nickel(II) complexes. *Organometallics* **2014**, *33*, 2012–2018. [CrossRef] [PubMed]
29. Armarego, W.L.F.; Chai, C.L.L. *Purification of Laboratory Chemicals*; Butterworth-Heinemann: Burlington, MA, USA, 2009.
30. Bruker. *APEX2 and SAINT*; Bruker AXS Inc.: Madison, WI, USA, 2014.
31. Sheldrick, G.M. Crystal structure refinement with SHELXL. *Acta Cryst. C* **2015**, *71*, 3–8. [CrossRef] [PubMed]
32. Frisch, M.J.; Trucks, G.W.; Schlegel, H.B.; Scuseria, G.E.; Robb, M.A.; Cheeseman, J.R.; Montgomery, J.A.; Kudin, K.N., Jr.; Burant, J.C.; Millam, J.M.; et al. *Gaussian 03, Revision E.01*; Gaussian Inc.: Wallingford, CT, USA, 2004.
33. Anufriev, S.A.; Sivaev, I.B.; Suponitsky, K.Y.; Godovikov, I.A.; Bregadze, V.I. Synthesis of 10-methylsulfide and 10-alkylmethylsulfonium *nido*-carborane derivatives: B-H$\cdots\pi$ Interactions between the B-H-B hydrogen atom and alkyne group in 10-RC≡CCH_2S(Me)-7,8-$C_2B_9H_{11}$. *Eur. J. Inorg. Chem.* **2017**, 4436–4443. [CrossRef]
34. Anufriev, S.A.; Sivaev, I.B.; Suponitsky, K.Y.; Bregadze, V.I. Practical synthesis of 9-methylthio-7,8-*nido*-carborane [9-MeS-7,8-$C_2B_9H_{11}]^-$. Some evidences of BH$\cdots$X hydride-halogen bonds in 9- XCH_2(Me)S-7,8-$C_2B_9H_{11}$ (X = Cl, Br, I). *J. Organomet. Chem.* **2017**, *849-850*, 315–323. [CrossRef]
35. Suponitsky, K.Y.; Tafur, S.; Masunov, A.E. Applicability of hybrid density functional theory methods to calculation of molecular hyperpolarizability. *J. Chem. Phys.* **2008**, *129*, 044109. [CrossRef]
36. Suponitsky, K.Y.; Masunov, A.E.; Antipin, M.Y. Conformational dependence of the first molecular hyperpolarizability in the computational design of nonlinear optical materials for optical switching. *Mendeleev. Commun.* **2008**, *18*, 265–267. [CrossRef]
37. Bader, R.F.W. *Atoms in Molecules. A Quantum Theory*; Clarendon Press: Oxford, UK, 1990.
38. Keith, T.A. *AIMAll (Version 15.05.18)*; TK Gristmill Software: Overland Park, KS, USA, 2015.
39. Espinosa, E.; Molins, E.; Lecomte, C. Hydrogen bond strengths revealed by topological analyses of experimentally observed electron densities. *Chem. Phys. Lett.* **1998**, *285*, 170–173. [CrossRef]
40. Espinosa, E.; Alkorta, I.; Rozas, I.; Elguero, J.; Molins, E. About the evaluation of the local kinetic, potential and total energy densities in closed-shell interactions. *Chem. Phys. Lett.* **2001**, *336*, 457–461. [CrossRef]
41. Lyssenko, K.A. Analysis of supramolecular architectures: Beyond molecular packing diagrams. *Mendeleev. Commun.* **2012**, *22*, 1–7. [CrossRef]
42. Suponitsky, K.Y.; Lyssenko, K.A.; Ananyev, I.V.; Kozeev, A.M.; Sheremetev, A.B. Role of weak intermolecular interactions in the crystal structure of tetrakis-furazano[3,4-c:3′,4′-g:3″,4″-k:3‴,4‴-o][1,2,5,6,9,10,13,14]octaazacyclohexadecine and its solvates. *Cryst. Growth Des.* **2014**, *14*, 4439–4449. [CrossRef]
43. Dmitrienko, A.O.; Karnoukhova, V.A.; Potemkin, A.A.; Struchkova, M.I.; Kryazhevskikh, I.A.; Suponitsky, K.Y. The influence of halogen type on structural features of compounds containing α-halo-α,α-dinitroethyl moieties. *Chem. Heterocycl. Comp.* **2017**, *53*, 532–539. [CrossRef]

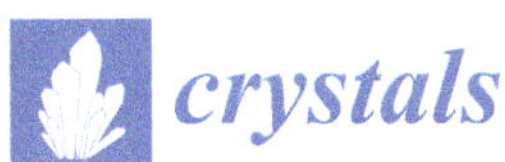

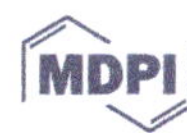

Article

Tuning the Liquid Crystallinity of Cholesteryl-*o*-Carborane Dyads: Synthesis, Structure, Photoluminescence, and Mesomorphic Properties

Albert Ferrer-Ugalde [1,†], Arántzazu González-Campo [1,†], José Giner Planas [1], Clara Viñas [1], Francesc Teixidor [1], Isabel M. Sáez [2,*] and Rosario Núñez [1,*,‡]

[1] Institut de Ciència de Materials de Barcelona, ICMAB-CSIC, Campus UAB, 08193 Bellaterra, Spain; a.ferrer80@hotmail.com (A.F.-U.); agonzalez@icmab.es (A.G.-C.); jginerplanas@icmab.es (J.G.P.); clara@icmab.es (C.V.); teixidor@icmab.es (F.T.)

[2] Agap Materials Solutions UK, Hull HU16 4RL, UK

* Correspondence: crapims1907@gmail.com (I.M.S.); rosario@icmab.es (R.N.)

† A.F.-U. and A.G.-C. contributed equally to this work.

‡ Dedicated to the Professor, friend and colleague Alan Welch who has managed with his research and enthusiasm at bringing boron cluster chemistry closer to the scientific community.

Abstract: A set of mesomorphic materials in which the *o*-carborane cluster is covalently bonded to a cholesteryl benzoate moiety (mesogen group) through a suitably designed linker is described. The olefin cross-metathesis between appropriately functionalized styrenyl-*o*-carborane derivatives and a terminal alkenyl cholesteryl benzoate mesogen (all type I terminal olefins) leads to the desired *trans*-regioisomer, which is the best-suited configuration to obtain mesomorphic properties in the final materials. The introduction of different substituents (R = H (**M2**), Me (**M3**), or Ph (**M4**)) to one of the carbon atoms of the *o*-carborane cluster ($C_{cluster}$) enables the tailoring of liquid crystalline properties. Compounds **M2** and **M3** show the chiral nematic (N*) phase, whereas **M4** do not show liquid crystal behavior. Weaker intermolecular interactions in the solid **M3** with respect to those in **M2** may allow the liquid crystallinity in **M3** to be expressed as enantiotropic behavior, whereas breaking the stronger intermolecular interaction in the solid state of **M2** leads directly to the isotropic state, resulting in monotropic behavior. Remarkably, **M3** also displays the blue phase, which was observed neither in the chiral nematic precursor nor in the styrenyl-cholesterol model (**M5**) without an *o*-carborane cluster, which suggests that the presence of the cluster plays a role in stabilizing this highly twisted chiral phase. In the carborane-containing mesogens (**M2** and **M3**), the *o*-carborane cluster can be incorporated without destroying the helical organization of the mesophase.

Keywords: boron clusters; carboranes; liquid crystals; fluorescence; cholesterol

Citation: Ferrer-Ugalde, A.; González-Campo, A.; Planas, J.G.; Viñas, C.; Teixidor, F.; Sáez, I.M.; Núñez, R. Tuning the Liquid Crystallinity of Cholesteryl-*o*-Carborane Dyads: Synthesis, Structure, Photoluminescence, and Mesomorphic Properties. *Crystals* **2021**, *11*, 133. https://doi.org/10.3390/cryst11020133

Academic Editor: Marina Yu. Stogniy
Received: 23 December 2020
Accepted: 24 January 2021
Published: 28 January 2021

1. Introduction

The liquid crystalline state (mesophase) is a state of matter that displays properties between those of conventional liquid and solid phases; this behavior can be subdivided into two types: thermotropic and lyotropic. Among these, thermotropic liquid crystals (LCs) are partially ordered anisotropic fluids that exhibit one or more mesophases in a given temperature range [1–3]. In most cases, the mesogenic behavior of an LC material is due to the combination of a rigid core with flexible groups to produce rod-like molecules that may show different types of mesophases, such as nematic (N) or smectic (Sm) [1]. Both the electronic structure and geometry determine the thermal and optical properties of the mesogen. Cholesteric liquid crystals (CLCs) are well-known chiral nematic materials that display the chiral nematic phase (N*), where the chiral molecules are organized in parallel planes to the director and twisted in a perpendicular way throughout the director, describing a helical structure. The most important feature of CLCs is the selective reflection of circularly polarized light according to Bragg's law [4]. Due to their 1D photonic structure and ease of fabrication, cholesteric liquid crystals have also attracted much attention as optical sensors [5–7].

Icosahedral 1,2-dicarba-*closo*-dodecacarborane or *o*-carborane (1,2-$C_2B_{10}H_{12}$) [8–11] have highly polarizable spherical aromaticity through σ-delocalized electron densities [12–16]. Consequently, they display characteristic electronic properties [17,18], and thermal [19–21], chemical, and photochemical stability [22,23]. All these features make them attractive and interesting systems in materials science [24–26], especially for luminescent materials [27–48], polymers [21], and Non-Linear Optical (NLO) materials, [49,50] among others [22]. The rigidity of these boron clusters promotes their use as a structural element of the rigid core in the preparation of liquid crystalline materials [51]. Boron clusters of major interest for synthesizing liquid crystals have been the 12 vertex, *p*-carborane (1,12-$C_2B_{10}H_{12}$) [52,53], $[1\text{-}CB_{11}H_{12}]^-$ [54–56], the dianion dodecaborate $[B_{12}H_{12}]^{2-}$ [57], as well as the 10 vertex *closo*-boron clusters 1,10-$C_2B_8H_{10}$, $[1\text{-}CB_9H_{10}]^-$ [54,58]. All of them are properly functionalized with suitable organic functional groups to provide a supramolecular structure with optical properties that might be modulated by external stimuli (Chart 1) [8]. Around 200 "rod-like" mesogens containing *p*-carboranes and several examples of bent-core mesogens bearing *m*-carborane (1,7-$C_2B_{10}H_{12}$) have been reported, in which the angle formed for both substituents at the carbons of the cluster ($C_{cluster}$, C_c) is 120° [51]. Generally, *p*-carboranes are the preferred choice to synthesize LCs, not only because of their spherocylindrical morphology, but also for the accessibility of substitution at the antipodal C_c atoms with appropriate groups, leading to an extension of the molecular shape that forms the mesogenic state (Chart 1). Most LCs containing *p*-carboranes show nematic phases [59], except those LCs with terminal alkyl chains with fluoride atoms that usually lead to smectic phases [60]. Nevertheless, the use of *o*-carborane, 1,2-$C_2B_{10}H_{12}$, and its derivatives has barely been explored as LCs, but studies involving their use in boron-containing liposomes as potential agents for BNCT have been reported [61–64]. To our knowledge, only two examples on *o*-carborane-based LCs have been recently reported by Kaszynsky [65,66]. In these, *o*-carborane is used as a linear structural element with a moderate dipole moment, which is substituted at the C1 and B12 atoms to give 1,12-difunctionalized derivatives that show the smectic A (SmA) and N mesophases.

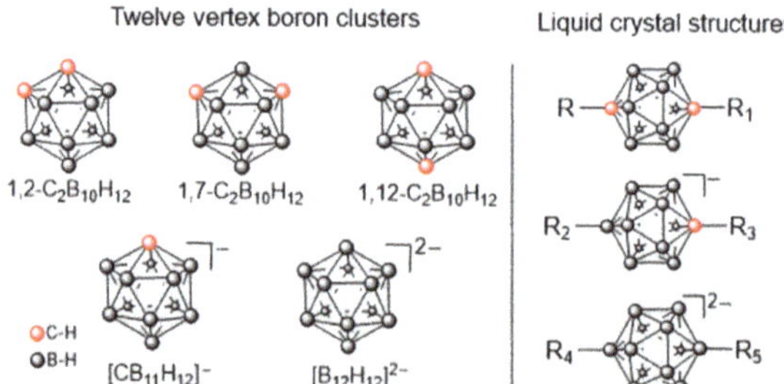

Chart 1. Representation of more usual twelve vertex boron clusters used to perform liquid crystalline materials.

There have been several reports of liquid crystals containing octasilsesquioxanes [67,68], or fullerenes [69–71], as scaffold to append mesogenic moieties in order to probe the effect of a rigid structurally well-defined core on mesophase behavior. In this sense, *o*-carborane may also provide a unique inorganic polyhedral scaffold that can lead the way to the generation of a new family of this class of materials, and it may offer a new insight into the effects of these substituents on the mesophase behavior of the ensuing liquid crystalline materials.

Herein we describe for the first time the synthesis, structural characterization, and photophysical properties in solution of a set of new mesomorphic materials in which the *o*-carborane cluster is covalently bonded to a cholesteryl benzoate moiety (mesogen group) through a suitable methylene linker. We have assessed the influence of the *o*-carborane unit and its substituents bound to the C_c atom on their liquid crystal properties. We have also tried to establish a relationship between the 3D crystal packing in solid state and the changes of mesophase with temperature.

2. Results and Discussion

2.1. Synthesis and Characterization of Mesogens

The chemical synthesis of linear cholesteryl-*o*-carborane dyads was designed to be carried out by olefin cross-metathesis between three different styrenyl-*o*-carborane derivatives: 1-[$CH_2C_6H_4$-4′-($CH=CH_2$)]-2-R-1,2-*closo*-$C_2B_{10}H_{10}$ [R = H (**1**), R = Methyl or Me (**2**), R = Phenyl or Ph (**3**)] (see Scheme 1) [42], and a cholesterol derivative that contains a suitable alkenylene moiety. To this purpose, cholesteryl benzoate was adequately modified to introduce the terminal alkenylene group producing **M1** by adaptation of the literature method (Scheme S1) [72]. A related strategy using olefin cross-metathesis in the design of liquid crystal synthesis has been reported while the current work was in progress [73,74]. Cross-metathesis reactions of *o*-carborane derivatives **1–3** and the mesogenic cholesterol derivative **M1** were carried out using first-generation Grubbs catalyst in CH_2Cl_2 at reflux for 48 h under argon atmosphere (Scheme 1). The reactions were by ^{1}H NMR spectroscopy to the total disappearance of the starting vinyl and alkenyl protons. The white solid in the remaining suspensions, which corresponds to the homo-metathesis of the **M1** side product, was filtered off, and the clear brown solutions were quenched with methanol to yield a gray precipitate that was also filtered and dried. Spectroscopic analyses proved that the latter contained a mixture of the expected final compound (**M2–M4**) and a small quantity of the **M1** homo-metathesis compound, which is partially soluble in CH_2Cl_2. Although we did not use excess of **1–3** to avoid the formation of compounds from their homo-metathesis, some of them were obtained and remained in the MeOH solution. The gray precipitates were finally purified by column chromatography affording the *o*-carborane-containing dyads **M2**, **M3**, and **M4** as white solids in 54, 50, and 49% yield, respectively.

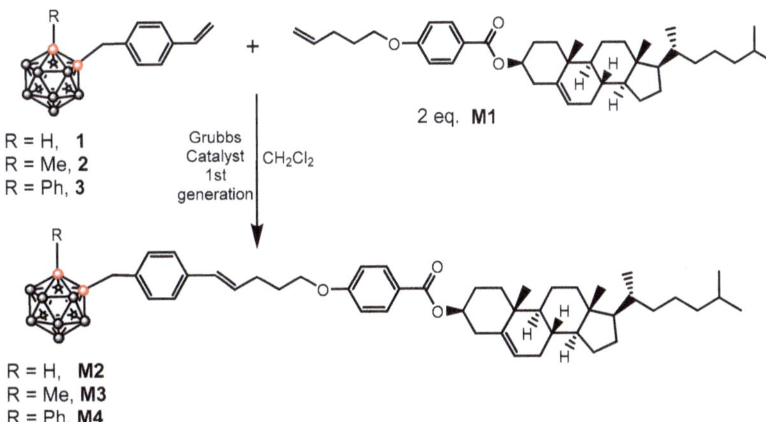

Scheme 1. Synthesis of cholesteryl-*o*-carborane dyads **M2–M4**.

In order to understand the influence of the *o*-carborane cluster and its substituent bound to the C_c atom on the mesogenic behavior of **M2–M4**, a carborane-free compound **M5** was also synthesized by cross-metathesis of pure styrene with the mesogen **M1** (Scheme 2). We used the same conditions as those for **M2–M4** with a large excess of styrene due to the ease of the styrene to give the compound from homo-metathesis. **M5** was isolated as a white solid in 82% yield after purification by column chromatography.

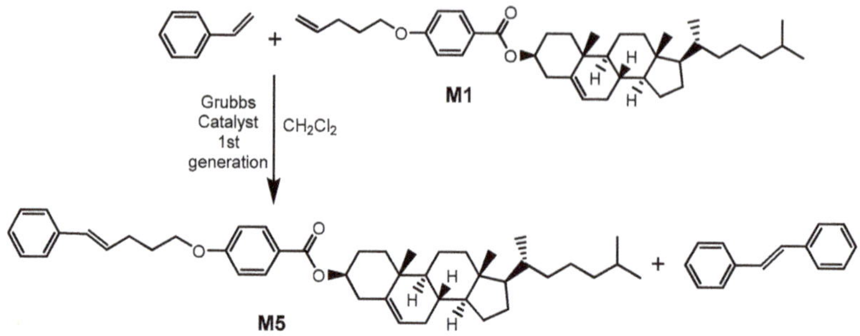

Scheme 2. Synthesis of carborane-free cholesterol derivative **M5**.

Complete cross-metathesis between **M1** with styrenyl-*o*-carborane derivatives **1–3** or styrene afforded **M2–M5**, which was confirmed by standard spectroscopy techniques such as FT-IR, ^{11}B, ^{1}H, and ^{13}C NMR, MALDI-TOF mass spectroscopy and elemental analysis. A detailed description of the characterization is included in the Supporting Information. In addition, suitable single crystals of **M2**, **M3**, and **M5** were analyzed by X-ray diffraction.

2.2. *X-Ray Crystal Structures of* **M2**, **M3**, *and* **M5**

Single crystals of **M2**, **M3**, and **M5** suitable for X-ray diffraction analysis were obtained by slow evaporation of CH_2Cl_2 (**M2–3**) or toluene (**M5**) solutions and found suitable for X-ray diffraction analysis. The molecular structures of **M2**, **M3**, and **M5** are shown in Figures 1 and 2. The main cell crystal parameters can be found in Table S1. A list of selected data and bonding parameters can also be found in the Supporting Information (Tables S2–S4).

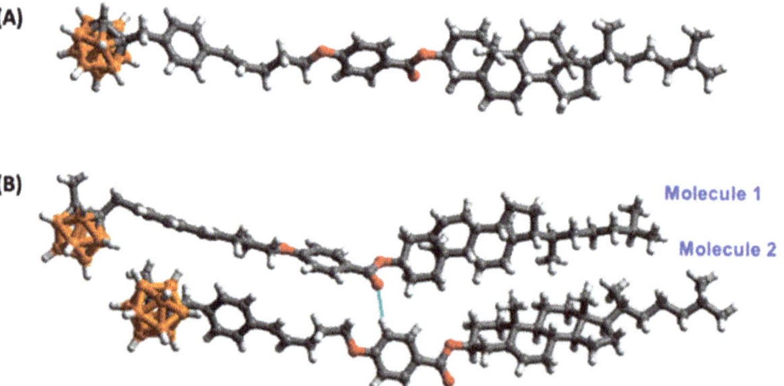

Figure 1. View of independent molecules in the unit cell of **M2** (**A**) and **M3** (**B**). Intermolecular contacts are shown as dotted blue lines. Color codes: H white; C gray; O red; B orange.

Whereas both *o*-carborane-containing dyads **M2** and **M3** crystallized in the monoclinic and non-centrosymmetric $P2_1$ space group, the styrene derivative **M5** crystallized in the triclinic *P1* space group. As shown in Figures 1 and 2 and Figures S16 and S17, unit cells for the compounds showed one, two, or four molecules of **M2**, **M3**, and **M5**, respectively. The shape of the molecules was similar, although slightly different geometries can be observed in **M3** (Figure 1) and **M5** (Figure 2). In particular, the angles between the plane of the benzoate and the steroid ring in **M3** (i.e., for the C2–C7 plane and C24–C28 mean plane) were 69.50(14)° and 55.15(16)°, respectively, and between the benzoate ring and the C_6H_4 ring close to the cluster (i.e., for the C2–C7 plane and C13–C18 plane), they were 25.77(14)° and 136.64(15), respectively.

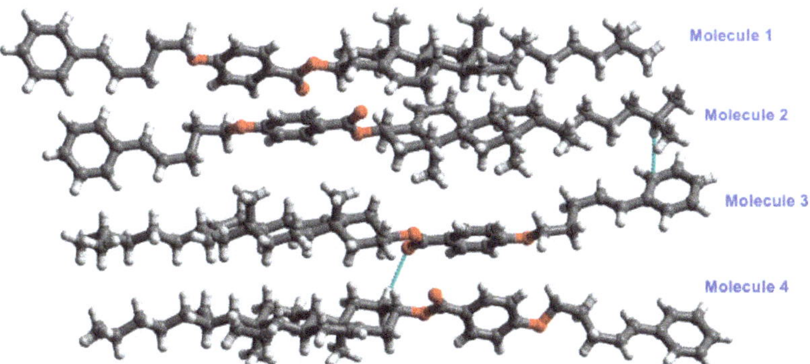

Figure 2. View of independent molecules in the unit cell of **M5**. Intermolecular contacts are shown as dotted blue lines. Color codes: H white; C gray; O red; B orange.

In general, the packing motifs in the crystals were similar for all structures. Indeed, the **M2**, **M3**, and **M5** structures were built from tilted molecules to form layers that were piled giving the observed 3D structures (Figure 3). In all cases, layers were formed by self-assembled molecules oriented parallel to each other (Figure S18). The densities of the 3D structures decreased in the order **M5** (1.152 g cm^{-3}) > **M3** (1.135 g cm^{-3}) > **M2** (1.122 g cm^{-3}).

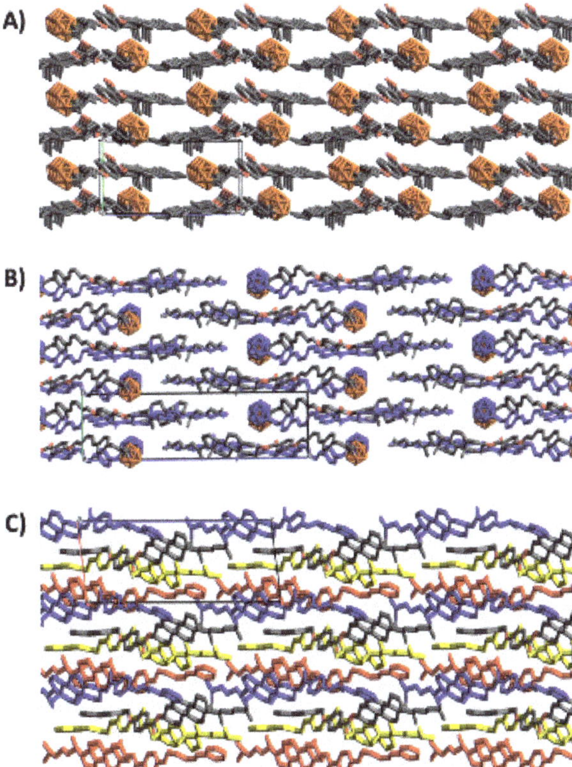

Figure 3. Views of crystal packings of **M2** (**A**), **M3** (**B**), and **M5** (**C**). Independent molecules in the unit cells are colored. H atoms are omitted for clarity.

As it is the case in a large majority of mesogens [73–75], and also in the case of most *o*-carborane derivatives [76], the molecules presented here have no strong hydrogen bond donor groups. Therefore, in the obtained crystals, molecules in the layers as well as interactions within the layers are stabilized by weak intermolecular interactions. This is clearly confirmed by the Hirshfeld surface analysis [77] for **M2**, **M3**, and **M5**. The analysis clearly showed the presence of weak H···H and H···O interactions, with no long sharp spikes characteristic of strong hydrogen bonds and the absence of strong π–π interactions in the Fingerprint plots (Figure S19) [78]. The relative contributions of different interactions to the Hirshfeld surface were calculated from the Fingerprint plots (Figure 4). From this simple analysis, it can be clearly observed that H/H contacts correspond to 78–84% of the total Hirshfeld surface area for these molecules, which is consistent with the large ratio of external H to N, O, or C atoms. C/H contacts comprise around 13–15% to the total Hirshfeld surface area and C/C (i.e., π–π) interactions contribute from 0.8% in the non-carborane derivative **M5** to an almost negligible percentage in the carborane compounds **M2** and **M3** (Figure 4).

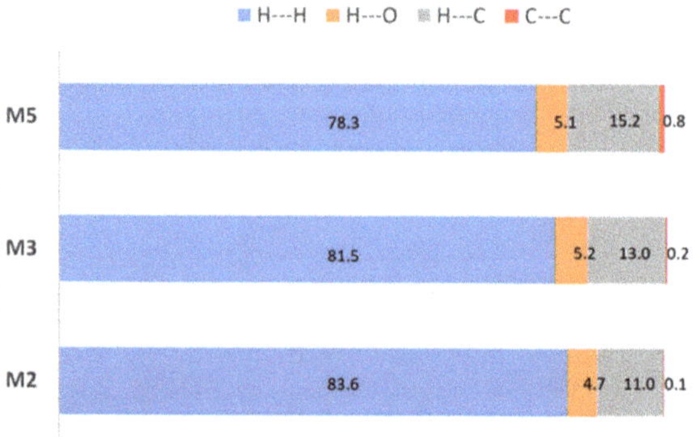

Figure 4. Relative contributions of various intermolecular contacts to the Hirshfeld surface area in all compounds in this study.

Analysis of the data in Figure 4 clearly indicated that the introduction of the *o*-carborane moieties into the mesogen **M1** increases the percentage of H···H contacts, while it decreases the percentage of H/C and C/C contacts. The decrease of the latter two is consistent with the spherical shape of *o*-carborane disrupting the supramolecular contacts of merely flat and aromatic systems (e.g., C–H···π and π–π), and this may affect the mesogenic properties of **M2** and **M3** when compared to **M5** (vide infra). In addition to this, spatial requirements for the carborane cages in these molecules disrupt the efficient packing that, in the absence of these spherical cages, is observed in rod-like molecules such as **M5** (Figure 3). This is experimentally observed in the calculated densities of the crystals for **M2**, **M3**, and **M5** (vide supra).

2.3. Photophysical Properties

The photophysical properties of **M2–M5**, including absorption and emission maxima (λ_{abs} and λ_{em}), fluorescence quantum yields (Φ_f), and Stokes shifts were assessed in CH_2Cl_2 (Figure S20 and Table 1). The UV-Vis spectra showed strong maximum absorption peaks at λ_{abs} = 260 nm for **M2–M4** and λ_{abs} = 257 nm for the non-carborane containing **M5**, and there were two additional very weak shoulders around 285 and 295 nm (Figure S20). The absorption peaks were attributed to the π–π* transitions of the styrenyl group, which is the fluorophore of the molecule, and they appear in the same region as that of the starting compounds **1–3** [42]. Compounds **M2**, **M3**, and **M5** displayed emission maxima at λ_{em} = 317 and 319 nm for **M2** and **M3** respectively, whereas **M5** exhibited a maximum at 315 nm after excitation at 260 nm (Figure S20). On the contrary, compound **M4** did not show fluorescence emission in solution. These results indicated that the emission properties of **M2–M4** were essentially the same as for their precursors **1–3**. In previous works, we demonstrated that the photoluminescence properties of precursors **1–3** and their derivatives were influenced by the substituents bound to the C_c atom [42], where it was proved that the Ph-*o*-carborane moiety acts as an electron-withdrawing group, leading to an efficient quenching of the fluorescence due to a charge transfer process [42,46]. This would explain the fluorescence quenching for **M4**. Fluorescence quantum yield values (Φ_f) confirmed that **M2** exhibited the highest efficiency (24.8%), whereas **M3** and **M5** displayed similar values to each other around 12.2%. It is noteworthy that compounds **M2–M4** followed the same trend for their emission properties than their respective precursors **1–3**. Noteworthy, the Stokes shift values did not vary significantly within the three luminescent compounds, being all of them close to the region of 7000 cm^{-1}.

Table 1. Photophysical properties of **M1–M5**.

Compound	λ_{abs} (nm)	λ_{em} (nm)	Φ_f (%)	Stokes Shift ($cm^{-1}/10^3$)
M1	266	-	-	-
M2	260	317	24.8	6.92
M3	260	319	12.2	7.11
M4	260	-	-	-
M5	257	315	12.1	7.16

All spectra were recorded in CH_2Cl_2. All samples were prepared to obtain an absorbance of around 0.1 at the excitation wavelength. Quantum yields Φ_f were calculated using quinine sulfate in a 0.5 M aqueous solution of H_2SO_4 ($\Phi_f = 0.54$) as a standard. Stokes shift = $-10^*(1/\lambda_{em} - 1/\lambda_{abs})$.

2.4. Liquid Crystal Properties

The mesomorphic properties of **M1–M5** were investigated by differential scanning calorimetry (DSC) and polarized optical microscopy (POM). The DSC thermograms of **M2–M5** are shown in Figures S21–S24, and the transition temperatures are listed in Table 2. Selected optical textures determined by POM are presented in Figure 5. The cross-metathesis reaction between the cholesteryl benzoate and the styrenyl-*o*-carborane derivatives produced only the *trans*-regioisomer, which is the preferred configuration to induce liquid crystallinity. The *o*-carborane derivative **M3** (R = Me) is the one that has the most attractive mesomorphic behavior. On cooling from the isotropic state, POM showed the presence of the rare blue phase over a very narrow temperature range (≈0.1 °C), which was identified by the mosaic texture (Figure 5b) with very low birefringence [79]. On further cooling, it was followed by the N* phase, which was identified by the Grandjean planar texture typical of the N* phase (Figure 5a). The blue phase could not be observed in the DSC thermogram, but the thermogram showed clearly the enantiotropic nature of the N* phase. Pleasingly, mesogens **M2** (R = H) and **M3** (R = Me) also displayed the N* phase, indicating that the N* phase of the cholesterol substituent was preserved upon attachment to the styrenyl-*o*-carborane cluster. The N* mesophase of **M3** is enantiotropic in nature (Figure 5a), whereas for **M2**, it is a monotropic N* phase. It is important to note that **M2** showed considerable supercooling of the transition from the isotropic state to the N* phase, as observed by DSC and POM. The alkenyl cholesteryl benzoate precursor **M1** showed a wide temperature range N*, from 131.4 °C (crystalline state) to 238 °C (isotropic liquid). The model compound **M5** showed the enantiotropic N* phase over a range ≈ 70 °C, with a clearing point at 224 °C (Figure 5d), which is at a lower temperature than **M1** (238 °C), indicating the slightly lower thermal stability of the mesophase in comparison with **M1** (Table 2). Interestingly, neither **M1** nor **M5** showed blue phase, suggesting that the *o*-carborane cluster plays a role in stabilizing the intermolecular interactions needed to support the blue phase. Comparison of the transition temperatures showed that the *o*-carborane-containing dyads **M2–M4** have lower isotropization temperatures than **M5** (Table 2). This comparison suggested that the presence of the spherical *o*-carborane cluster disrupts significantly the intermolecular interactions of the cholesteryl benzoate cores needed to induce the mesophase. The higher isotropization temperature of **M2** in comparison with **M3** indicated stronger intermolecular interactions in **M2** (R = H) than in **M3** (R = Me). The introduction of an Me group at the *o*-carborane cluster adds steric hindrance and makes space filling more difficult, resulting in a lower clearing point. This different mesogenic behavior between **M2** and **M3** could be rationalized, taking into account the differences between the solid state at room temperature and the liquid crystalline state, if we consider that the number of H···H contacts in the 3D crystal packing of **M2** is higher than in **M3** confirmed by the Hirshfeld surface analysis (vide supra). In contrast, both mesophase range and stability of **M5**, without the *o*-carborane moiety, are higher than those for **M2** and **M3**. A similar volume effect has been observed when carbocyclic moieties are used as end-groups in certain mesogens [80]. This might be related to the disrupting effect of the *o*-carborane cluster on the N* phase. On the other hand, *o*-carborane derivative **M4** (R = Ph) did not show liquid crystallinity, only a series of crystal forms, despite the presence of the strongly nematogen substituent. In this case, the presence of the phenyl group at the *o*-carborane cluster led to a largely bent geometry that disrupts any intermolecular interactions of the cholesterol rigid core needed to promote mesogenic behavior. This is supported by the melting point of **M4**, which was the lowest of the three cholesteryl-*o*-carborane derivatives.

Table 2. Phase transition temperatures (°C) and corresponding enthalpy values (J mol^{-1}, in square brackets) obtained from differential scanning calorimetry (DSC) second heating cycles for compounds **M2–M5**.

Compound	Phase Transition Temperatures (°C) and Enthalpy Values (J·mol^{-1})
M1	Cr 131.4 [27.3] N* 238.6 [1.3] Iso liq.
M2	g 53.1 [2.0] (N* 134.9 [−10.1]) Cr_2 181.7 [−2.9] Iso liq.
M3	g 47.9 [2.1] Cr_1 87.1 [−13.2] Cr_2 161.6 [22.0] N* 176.2 [2.1] (BP) Iso liq.
M4	g 22.6 [2.7] Cr_1 86.2 [−1.6] Cr_2 151.9 [29.3] Iso liq.
M5	Cr 150.2 [47.8] N* 224.2 [3.7] Iso liq.

N*: chiral nematic phase.

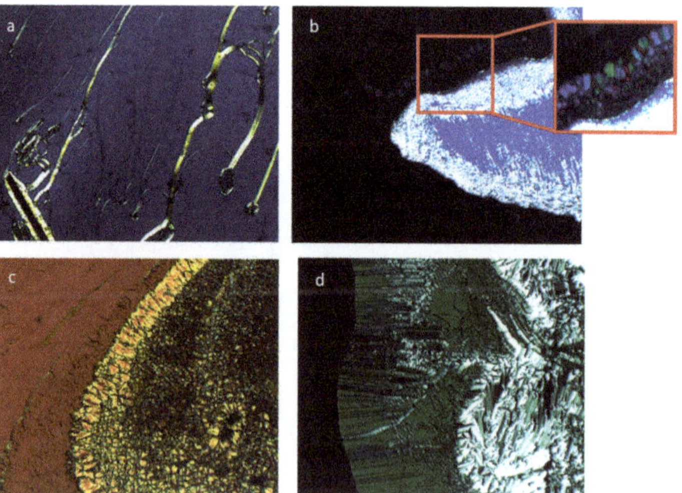

Figure 5. (**a**) Optical texture of **M3** in the N* phase at 162.2 °C. (**b**) Polarized optical microscopy (POM) image of the blue phase of **M3**. (**c**) POM image of **M2** at 119.0 °C on cooling from the isotropic liquid, showing the N* and crystal phases. (**d**) POM image of **M5** at 186.2 °C during the cooling cycle showing the N* phase.

Remarkably, these results indicated that the mesomorphic properties of cholesteryl-*o*-carborane dyads **M2–M4** could be modulated by modifying the substituent at the adjacent C_c atom. Non-substituted (**M2**) and Me-substituted **M3** displayed liquid crystals properties, whereas **M4** bearing a Ph group did not show liquid crystallinity. This suggested that the *o*-carborane is a suitable platform for liquid crystals and also may enable tuning of the liquid crystals properties of an attached mesogen group.

3. Materials and Methods

3.1. Materials

All reactions were performed under an atmosphere of argon employing standard Schlenk techniques. Anhydrous dichloromethane was purchased from Aldrich and used as received. 1-[$CH_2C_6H_4$-4′-(CH=CH_2)]-2-H-1,2-*closo*-$C_2B_{10}H_{10}$ (**1**), 1-[$CH_2C_6H_4$-4′-(CH=CH_2)]-2-CH_3-1,2-*closo*-$C_2B_{10}H_{10}$ (**2**), and 1-[$CH_2C_6H_4$-4′-(CH=CH_2)]-2-C_6H_5-1,2-*closo*-$C_2B_{10}H_{10}$ (**3**) were obtained as described in the literature [42]. **M1** was prepared according to the literature process [72]. Reagent grade styrene and first generation Grubbs catalyst were purchased from Aldrich (St. Louis, MO, USA) and used as received. Solvents and all other reagents were purchased from Aldrich and used as received. Reactions were monitored by thin layer chromatography (TLC) using an appropriate solvent system. Silica-coated aluminium TLC plates used were purchased from Merck, Kenilworth, NJ, USA (Kieselgel 60 F-254) and visualized using either UV light (254 nm and 365 nm), or by oxidation with either iodine or aqueous potassium permanganate solution.

3.2. Instrumentation

Infrared spectra were measured on a Perkin-Elmer Spectrum 400 FT-IR/FT FIR (Waltham, MA, USA) and Shimadzu IR Prestige-21 (Kyoto, Japan) with Specac Golden Gate diamond ATR IR insert (Orpington, UK). ^{1}H NMR (300.13 MHz and 400 MHz) and $^{13}C\{^{1}H\}$ NMR spectra (75.47 MHz, 100.5 MHz) were obtained using Varian Unity Inova 400 MHz (Palo Alto, CA, USA), JEOL ECX 400 MHz (Akishima, Tokyo, Japan) and Bruker ARX 300 spectrometers (Billerica, MA, USA). The $^{11}B\{^{1}H\}$ NMR spectra (96.29 MHz) were run on a Bruker ARX 300 spectrometer. All experiments were made with concentrations between 15 and 20 mg/mL at 25 °C. Chemical shifts (ppm) are relative to $Si(CH_3)_4$ for ^{1}H (of residual proton; δ 7.25 ppm) and $^{13}C\{^{1}H\}$ NMR (δ 77.23 ppm signal) in $CDCl_3$. Chemical shift values for $^{11}B\{^{1}H\}$ NMR spectra were referenced to external $BF_3{\cdot}OEt_2$. Chemical shifts are reported in units of parts per million downfield from the reference, and all coupling constants are reported in Hz. Mass spectra were recorded on a Bruker Solarix FT-ICR (MALDI TOF/TOF™ spectra). UV/Vis spectra were measured on a Perkin Elmer Lambda 900 and Shimadzu UV-1700 Pharmaspec spectrophotometers using 1.0 cm cuvettes. Fluorescence emission spectra were recorded in a Perkin-Elmer LS-45 (230 V) Fluorescence spectrometer. Samples were prepared in spectroscopic grade solvents and adjusted to a response within the linear range. No fluorescent contaminants were detected on excitation in the wavelength region of experimental interest. CHN Elemental analyses were performed using an Exeter Analytical Inc. CE440 analyzer (North Chelmsford, MA, USA).

3.3. X-ray Diffraction

Diffraction data were collected at 110 K on an Oxford Diffraction SuperNova diffractometer (Abingdon, Oxfordshire, UK) with Mo-K_α radiation (λ = 0.71073 Å) using an EOS CCD camera (Canon, Tokyo, Japan). The crystal was cooled with an Oxford Instruments Cryojet. Diffractometer control, data collection, initial unit cell determination, frame integration, and unit-cell refinement was carried out with "Crysalis" [81]. Face-indexed absorption corrections were applied using spherical harmonics, implemented in a SCALE3 ABSPACK scaling algorithm [81]. OLEX2c was used for overall structure solution, refinement, and preparation of computer graphics and publication data. Within OLEX2, the algorithm used for structure solution was direct methods [82] for **M2** and **M3** and charge-flipping [83] for **M5**. Refinement by full-matrix least-squares used the SHELXL [82] algorithm within OLEX2 [84]. All non-hydrogen atoms were refined anisotropically. Hydrogen atoms were placed using a "riding model" and included in the refinement at calculated positions.

In the case of compound **M5**, the differences among molecules in the unit cell differ in the orientation of the steroid system, the benzoate, and the terminal phenyl ring. For the four molecules, the angle between the plane of the benzoate and the steroid ring was (50.71(12)°, 68.7(3)°, 54.87(13)°, and 40.88(12)°, respectively; the angle between the benzoate ring and the phenyl ring was 112.52(12)°, 93.8(3)°, 67.33(12)°, and 80.6(5)°, respectively. Two of the molecules exhibited disorder. For one, the benzoate ring and the *para*-OCH_2 was modeled in two positions with refined occupations of 0.684:0.316(4), whilst for the other, the phenyl was modeled in two positions with refined occupancies of 0.654:0.346(4). When calculating the planes for the angles described above, an average position was used.

3.4. *Phase Identification by Optical and Thermal Methods*

Polarized optical microscopy was performed on a Zeiss Axioskop 40Pol microscope (Oberkochen, Germany) using a Mettler FP82HT hotstage (Columbus, OH, USA) controlled by a Mettler FP90 central processor. Photomicrographs were captured via either an InfinityX-21 digital camera or a Sony NEX 5R mirrorless digital camera (Tokyo, Japan) mounted atop the microscope. Differential scanning calorimetry was performed on a Mettler DSC822e fitted with an autosampler operating with MettlerStar®software and calibrated before use against an indium standard (onset = 156.55 ± 0.2 °C, $\Delta H = 28.45 \pm 0.40\ Jg^{-1}$) under an atmosphere of dry nitrogen.

3.5. *Synthesis of Mesogens* **M2–M5**

3.5.1. Synthesis of **M2**

In a dry-oven 25 mL schlenk flask, 1-[$CH_2C_6H_4$-4′-(CH=CH_2)]-2-H-1,2-*closo*-$C_2B_{10}H_{10}$ (**1**) (68 mg, 0.26 mmol), **M1** (300 mg, 0.52 mmol), and first-generation Grubbs' catalyst (21 mg, 0.026 mmol) were dissolved in CH_2Cl_2 (10 mL). The solution was stirred and refluxed for 48 h. The reaction was monitored by ^1H NMR to the disappearance of the alkene protons of **M1**. After that, the mixture was cooled down to room temperature, filtered, and the brown solution was quenched by precipitation into 40 mL of methanol to afford a gray solid. This is filtered and purified by silica gel column chromatography (75% CH_2Cl_2–25% hexane), leading to compound **M2** as a pure white solid. Yield: 114 mg, 54%. A CH_2Cl_2 solution of **M2** gave crystals suitable for X-ray analysis. ^1H NMR ($CDCl_3$, TMS), δ (ppm): 7.97 (d, ^3J(H,H) = 8 Hz, 2H, C_6H_4), 7.30 (d, ^3J(H,H) = 8 Hz, 2H, C_6H_4), 7.05 (d, ^3J(H,H) = 8 Hz, 2H, C_6H_4), 6.89 (d, ^3J(H,H) = 8 Hz, 2H, C_6H_4), 6.40 (d, ^3J(H,H) = 16 Hz, 1H, C_6H_4CH=CH), 6.26 (dt, ^3J(H,H) = 16 Hz, ^3J(H,H) = 8 Hz, 1H, C_6H_4CH=*CH*), 5.40 (d, ^3J(H,H) = 6 Hz, 1H, (C_h)*CH*=CH), 4.81 (m, 1H, O*CH* (C_h)), 4.05 (t, 2H, ^3J(H,H) = 6 Hz, CH_2O), 3.48 (s, 2H, C_c-CH_2), 3.19 (s, 1H, C_c-*H*), 2.42 (m, 4H, $OCHCH_2$ (C_h) + C_6H_4CH=$CHCH_2$), 1.05 (s, 3H, C-CH_3), 0.91 (d, ^3J(H,H) = 6 Hz, 3H, $CHCH_3$), 0.85 (dd, ^3J(H,H) = 6 Hz, ^3J(H,H) = 3 Hz, 6H, $CH(CH_3)_2$), 0.67 (s, 3H, C-CH_3). $^{11}B\{^1H\}$ NMR ($CDCl_3$, $BF_3{\cdot}Et_2O$), δ (ppm): −3.33 (1B), −6.48 (1B), −9.90 (2B), −11.54 ppm (2B), −14.05 (4B). $^{13}C\{^1H\}$ NMR ($CDCl_3$, TMS), δ (ppm): 165.87 (s, C=O), 162.71 (s, C_{ar}-O), 139.84 (s, C=CH (C_h)), 137.84 (s, C_6H_4), 132.92 (s, C_6H_4), 131.62 (s, C_6H_4), 130.79 (s, C_6H_4), 130.08 (s, C_6H_4CH=CH), 129.93 (s, C_6H_4CH=CH), 126.62 (s, C_6H_4), 123.29 (s, C_6H_4), 122.78 (s, C_6H_4), 114.06 (s, C=CH (C_h)), 74.32 (s, CH-O), 67.31 (s, CH_2-O), 56.78 (s, CH (C_p)), 56.21 (s, CH (C_p)), 50.12 (s, CH (C_h)), 43.22 (s, CH (C_p-C_h)), 42.41 (s, C_c-CH_2), 39.83 (s, $CH_2CH(CH_3)_2$), 39.60 (s, CH (C_h)), 38.38 (s, CH_2C-O), 37.14 (s, CH (C_h)), 36.74 (s, CH (C_h)), 36.27 (s, CH_3CHCH_2), 35.89 (s, CH_3CHCH_2), 32.02 (s, CH (C_h)), 31.97 (s, CH (C_h)), 28.79 (s, CH=$CHCH_2CH_2$), 28.33 (s, CH (C_h)), 28.11 (s, CH (C_p)), 28.03 (s, CH-$(CH_3)_2$), 24.38 (s, CH_2 (C_p)), 26.90 (s, CH (C_h)), 24.38 (s, CH_2CH_2CH-$(CH_3)_2$), 23.92 (s, CH (C_h)), 22.92 (s, CH-$(CH_3)_2$), 22.66 (s, CH-$(CH_3)_2$), 21.13 (s, CH (C_h)), 19.48 (s, CH-CH_3), 18.81 (s, CH-CH_3), 11.95 ppm (s, CH-CH_3). ATR (cm^{-1}): 2939 (br s, C-H st), 2576 (br s, B-H st), 1697 (s, C=O st), 1604 (m,

C=C st). MALDI-TOF-MS (m/z): Calcd: 808.66. Found: 846.55 [M + K^+]. Anal. Calcd. for $C_{48}H_{74}B_{10}O_3$: C, 71.42; H, 9.24. Found: C, 71.58; H, 9.15.

3.5.2. Synthesis of **M3**

Compound **M3** was synthesized using the same procedure as for **M2**, but using 1-[$CH_2C_6H_4$-4′-(CH=CH_2)]-2-CH_3-1,2-*closo*-$C_2B_{10}H_{10}$ (**2**) (23 mg, 0.08 mmol), **M1** (100 mg, 0.17 mmol) and first-generation Grubbs catalyst (7 mg, 0.008 mmol) in 10 mL of CH_2Cl_2. After work-up, **M3** was obtained as a pure white solid. Yield: 38 mg, 50%. A CH_2Cl_2 solution of **M3** gave crystals suitable for X-ray analysis. ^{1}H NMR ($CDCl_3$, TMS), δ (ppm): 7.97 (d, ^{3}J(H,H) = 8 Hz, 2H, C_6H_4), 7.30 (d, ^{3}J(H,H) = 8 Hz, 2H, C_6H_4), 7.10 (d, ^{3}J(H,H) = 8 Hz, 2H, C_6H_4), 6.90 (d, ^{3}J(H,H) = 8 Hz, 2H, C_6H_4), 6.41 (d, ^{3}J(H,H) = 16 Hz, 1H, C_6H_4*CH*=CH), 6.25 (dt, ^{3}J(H,H) = 16 Hz, ^{3}J(H,H) = 6 Hz, 1H, C_6H_4CH=*CH*), 5.40 (d, ^{3}J(H,H) = 6 Hz, 1H, (C_h)*CH*=CH), 4.81 (m, 1H, O*CH* (C_h)), 4.05 (t, 2H, ^{3}J(H,H) = 6 Hz, CH_2O), 3.42 (s, 2H, C_c-CH_2), 2.42 (m, 4H, OCHCH_2 (C_h) + C_6H_4CH=CHCH_2), 2.14 (s, 3H, C_c-CH_3), 1.06 (s, 3H, C-CH_3), 0.91 (d, ^{3}J(H,H) = 6 Hz, 3H, CHCH_3), 0.85 (dd, ^{3}J(H,H) = 6 Hz, ^{3}J(H,H) = 3 Hz, 6H, CH(CH_3)$_2$), 0.67 (s, 3H, C-CH_3). ^{11}B{^{1}H} NMR ($CDCl_3$, BF_3·Et_2O), δ (ppm): −4.99 (1B), −6.55 (1B), −10.65 (4B), −11.29 ppm (4B). ^{13}C{^{1}H} NMR ($CDCl_3$, TMS), δ (ppm): 165.84 (s, C=O), 162.73 (s, C_{ar}-O), 139.86 (s, C=CH (C_h)), 137.38 (s, C_6H_4), 133.75 (s, C_6H_4), 131.60 (s, C_6H_4), 130.56 (s, C_6H_4), 130.35 (s, C_6H_4CH=CH), 130.11 (s, C_6H_4CH=CH), 126.20 (s, C_6H_4), 122.71 (s, C_6H_4), 114.01 (s, C=CH (C_h)), 74.27 (s, CH-O), 67.36 (s, CH_2-O), 56.78 (s, CH (C_p)), 56.21 (s, CH (C_p)), 50.12 (s, CH (C_h)), 42.40 (s, CH (C_p-C_h)), 41.01 (s, C_c-CH_2), 39.82 (s, CH_2CH(CH_3)$_2$), 39.60 (s, CH (C_h)), 38.38 (s, CH_2C-O), 37.14 (s, CH (C_h)), 36.74 (s, CH (C_h)), 36.27 (s, CH_3CHCH_2), 35.89 (s, CH_3CHCH_2), 32.02 (s, CH (C_h)), 31.97 (s, CH (C_h)), 29.47 (s, CH=CH$CH_2$$CH_2$), 28.82 (s, CH=CH$CH_2$$CH_2$), 28.33 (s, CH ($C_h$)), 28.11 (s, CH ($C_p$)), 28.03 (s, CH-($CH_3$)$_2$), 24.38 (s, CH_2 (C_p)), 23.91 (s, $CH_2$$CH_2$CH-($CH_3$)$_2$), 23.78 (s, C_c-CH_3), 22.92 (s, CH-(CH_3)$_2$), 22.66 (s, CH-(CH_3)$_2$), 21.13 (s, CH (C_h)), 19.48 (s, CH-CH_3), 18.81 (s, CH-CH_3), 11.95 ppm (s, CH-CH_3). ATR (cm^{-1}): 2931 (br s, C-H st), 2584 (br s, B-H st), 1705 (s, C=O st), 1604 (m, C=C st). MALDI-TOF-MS (m/z): Calcd: 822.67. Found: 860.56 [M + K^+]. Anal. Calcd. for $C_{49}H_{76}B_{10}O_3$: C, 71.66; H, 9.33. Found: C, 72.11; H, 9.32.

3.5.3. Synthesis of **M4**

Compound **M4** was synthesized using the same procedure as for **M2** and **M3** but using 1-[$CH_2C_6H_4$-4′-(CH=CH_2)]-2-C_6H_5-1,2-*closo*-$C_2B_{10}H_{10}$ (**3**) (50 mg, 0.15 mmol), **M1** (171 mg, 0.30 mmol) and first-generation Grubbs catalyst (12 mg, 0.015 mmol) in 6 mL of CH_2Cl_2. After work-up, **M4** was obtained as a pure white solid. Yield: 64 mg, 49%. ^{1}H NMR ($CDCl_3$, TMS), δ (ppm): 7.99 (d, ^{3}J(H,H) = 8 Hz, 2H, C_6H_4), 7.71 (d, ^{3}J(H,H) = 8 Hz, 2H, C_6H_5), 7.54–7.44 (m, 3H, C_6H_5), 7.20 (d, ^{3}J(H,H) = 8 Hz, 2H, C_6H_4), 7.10 (d, ^{3}J(H,H) = 8 Hz, 2H, C_6H_4), 6.90 (d, ^{3}J(H,H) = 8 Hz, 2H, C_6H_4), 6.75 (d, ^{3}J(H,H) = 8 Hz, 2H, C_6H_4), 6.38 (d, ^{3}J(H,H) = 16 Hz, 1H, C_6H_4CH=*CH*), 6.23 (dt, ^{3}J(H,H) = 16 Hz, ^{3}J(H,H) = 6 Hz, 1H, C_6H_4CH=*CH*), 5.41 (d, ^{3}J(H,H) = 6 Hz, 1H, (C_h)*CH*=CH), 4.83 (m, 1H, O*CH* (C_h)), 4.05 (t, 2H, ^{3}J(H,H) = 6 Hz, CH_2O), 3.04 (s, 2H, C_c-CH_2), 2.42 (m, 4H, OCHCH_2 (C_h) + C_6H_4CH=CHCH_2), 0.91 (d, ^{3}J(H,H) = 6 Hz, 3H, CHCH_3), 0.86 (dd, ^{3}J(H,H) = 6 Hz, ^{3}J(H,H) = 3 Hz, 6H, CH(CH_3)$_2$), 0.68 (s, 3H, C-CH_3). ^{11}B{^{1}H} NMR ($CDCl_3$, BF_3·Et_2O), δ (ppm): −4.39 (2B), −10.92 (8B); ^{13}C{^{1}H} NMR ($CDCl_3$, TMS), δ (ppm): 165.87 (s, C=O), 162.74 (s, C_{ar}-O), 139.86 (s, C=CH (C_h)), 137.15 (s, C_6H_4), 133.99 (s, C_6H_4), 131.62 (s, C_6H_4), 131.59 (s, C_6H_5), 130.93 (s, C_6H_5), 130.91 (s, C_6H_5), 130.56 (s, C_6H_4), 130.31 (s, C_6H_4CH=CH), 130.21 (s, C_6H_4), 130.10 (s, C_6H_4CH=CH), 129.13 (s, C_6H_5), 125.96 (s, C_6H_4), 123.26 (s, C_6H_4), 122.77 (s, C_6H_4), 114.07 (s, C=CH (C_h)), 83.76 (s, C_c-C_6H_5), 82.19 (s, Cc-CH_2), 74.30 (s, CH-O), 67.34 (s, CH_2-O), 56.79 (s, CH (C_p)), 56.22 (s, CH (C_p)), 50.13 (s, CH (C_h)), 42.41 (s, CH (C_p-C_h)), 40.72 (s, Cc-CH_2), 39.83 (s, CH_2CH(CH_3)$_2$), 39.61 (s, CH (C_h)), 38.39 (s, CH_2C-O), 37.15 (s, CH (C_h)), 36.75 (s, CH (C_h)), 36.28 (s, CH_3CHCH_2), 35.90 (s, CH_3CHCH_2), 32.03 (s, CH (C_h)), 31.97 (s, CH (C_h)), 29.46 (s, CH=CH$CH_2$$CH_2$), 28.82 (s, CH=CH$CH_2$$CH_2$), 28.34 (s, CH ($C_h$)), 28.11 (s, CH ($C_p$)), 28.04 (s, CH-($CH_3$)$_2$), 24.39 (s, CH_2 (C_p)), 23.93 (s, $CH_2$$CH_2$CH-($CH_3$)$_2$), 22.93 (s, CH-($CH_3$)$_2$), 22.67 (s, CH-($CH_3$)$_2$), 21.15 (s, CH ($C_h$)), 19.49 (s, CH-$CH_3$), 18.82 (s,

CH-CH_3), 11.96 (s, CH-CH_3). ATR (cm^{-1}): 2939 (br s, C-H st), 2584 (br s, B-H st), 1705 (s, C=O st), 1604 (m, C=C st). MALDI-TOF-MS (*m/z*): Calcd: 882.64. Found: 921.57 [M + K^+]. Anal. Calcd. for $C_{54}H_{78}B_{10}O_3$: C, 73.43; H, 8.90. Found: C, 72.89; H, 8.92.

3.5.4. Synthesis of **M5**

Compound **M5** was synthesized using the same procedure as for **M2**, but using styrene (0.5 mL 5.3 mmol), **M1** (100 mg, 0.17 mmol) and first-generation Grubbs catalyst (20 mg, 0.024 mmol) were dissolved in CH_2Cl_2 (5 mL). After work-up, **M5** was obtained as a pure white solid. Yield: 93 mg, 82%. A toluene solution of **M5** gave crystals suitable for X-ray analysis. ^{1}H NMR ($CDCl_3$, TMS), δ (ppm): 7.97 (d, ^{3}J(H,H) = 8 Hz, 2H, C_6H_4), 7.35–7.15 (m, 5H, C_6H_5), 6.90 (d, ^{3}J(H,H) = 8 Hz, 2H, C_6H_4), 6.43 (d, ^{3}J(H,H) = 12 Hz, 1H, C_6H_4*CH*=CH), 6.23 (dt, ^{3}J(H,H) = 12 Hz, ^{3}J(H,H) = 4.5 Hz, 1H, C_6H_4CH=*CH*), 5.40 (d, ^{3}J(H,H) = 6 Hz, 1H, (C_h)*CH*=CH), 4.81 (m, 1H, O*CH* (C_h)), 4.05 (t, 2H, ^{3}J(H,H) = 6 Hz, CH_2O), 2.42 (m, 2H, OCHCH_2 (C_h)), 1.06 (s, 3H, C-CH_3), 0.91 (d, ^{3}J(H,H) = 6 Hz, 3H, CHCH_3), 0.85 (dd, ^{3}J(H,H) = 6 Hz, ^{3}J(H,H) = 3 Hz, 6H, CH(CH_3)$_2$), 0.67 (s, 3H, C-CH_3). ^{13}C {^{1}H} NMR ($CDCl_3$, TMS), δ (ppm): 165.89 (s, C=O), 162.77 (s, C_{ar}-O), 139.86 (s, C=CH (C_h)), 137.60 (s, C_6H_5), 131.60 (s, C_6H_4), 130.89 (s, C_6H_5), 129.48 (s, C_6H_5), 128.60 (s, C_6H_5), 127.14 (s, C_6H_5), 126.20 (s, C_6H_5), 123.22 (s, C_6H_4), 122.71 (s, C_6H_4), 114.01 (s, C=CH (C_h)), 74.27 (s, CH-O), 67.36 (s, CH_2-O), 56.78 (s, CH (C_p)), 56.21 (s, CH (C_p)), 50.12 (s, CH (C_h)), 42.40 (s, CH (C_p-C_h)), 39.82 (s, CH_2CH(CH_3)$_2$), 39.60 (s, CH (C_h)), 38.38 (s, CH_2C-O), 37.14 (s, CH (C_h)), 36.74 (s, CH (C_h)), 36.27 (s, CH_3CHCH_2), 35.89 (s, CH_3CHCH_2), 32.02 (s, CH (C_h)), 31.97 (s, CH (C_h)), 29.47 (s, CH=CH$CH_2$$CH_2$), 28.82 (s, CH=CH$CH_2$$CH_2$), 28.33 (s, CH ($C_h$)), 28.11 (s, CH ($C_p$)), 28.03 (s, CH-($CH_3$)$_2$), 24.38 (s, CH_2 (C_p)), 23.91 (s, $CH_2$$CH_2$CH-($CH_3$)$_2$), 22.92 (s, CH-($CH_3$)$_2$), 22.66 (s, CH-($CH_3$)$_2$), 21.13 (s, CH ($C_h$)), 19.48 (s, CH-$CH_3$), 18.81 (s, CH-$CH_3$), 11.95 ppm (s, CH-$CH_3$). ATR ($cm^{-1}$): 2931 (br s, C-H st), 1697 (s, C=O st), 1604 (m, C=C st). MALDI-TOF-MS (*m/z*): Calcd: 650.47. Found: 673.46 [M + Na^+]. Anal. Calcd. for $C_{45}H_{62}O_3$: C, 83.03; H, 9.60. Found: C, 81.92; H, 9.55. (+1/2 MeOH $C_{45.5}H_{64}O_{3.5}$: C, 81.99; H, 9.60).

4. Conclusions

In conclusion, the olefin cross-metathesis between suitably substituted *o*-carborane derivatives and a mesogenic precursor as the modified cholesterol offers a strategy to obtain liquid crystalline materials. The reaction of styrenyl-*o*-carborane derivatives with a terminal alkenyl cholesteryl benzoate yields only the desired *trans*-regioisomer, which is the best-suited configuration to attain mesogenic behavior. The substituent linked to the C_c atom of the *o*-carborane plays an important role in tuning the liquid crystal behavior; for non-substituted *o*-carborane (**M2**, R = H) and methyl-substituted *o*-carborane (**M3**, R = Me), the N* phase was obtained, whereas **M4** (R = Ph) was not mesogenic. In addition, **M3** exhibited blue phase, which was observed neither in the chiral nematic precursor **M1** nor in the model compound **M5**, which suggested that the presence of the *o*-carborane cluster leads to stabilizing this highly twisted chiral phase in this set of compounds. In these cases, although the thermal stability and the range of the N* phase is substantially decreased in comparison with the precursors, the *o*-carborane cluster can be incorporated without destroying the helical organization of the mesophase.

Supplementary Materials: The following are available online at https://www.mdpi.com/2073-4352/11/2/133/s1. Scheme S1. Synthesis of the mesogen **M1**, Figure S1. ^{1}H-NMR of compound **M2**, Figure S2. ^{11}B{^{1}H}-NMR of compound **M2**, Figure S3. ^{13}C{^{1}H}-NMR of compound **M2**, Figure S4. ^{1}H-NMR of compound **M3, Figure S5.** ^{11}B{^{1}H}-NMR of compound **M3, Figure S6.** ^{13}C{^{1}H}-NMR of compound **M3**, Figure S7. ^{1}H-NMR of compound **M4**, Figure S8. ^{11}B{^{1}H}-NMR of compound **M4**, Figure S9. ^{13}C{^{1}H}-NMR of compound **M4**, Figure S10. ^{1}H-NMR of compound **M5**, Figure S11. ^{13}C{^{1}H}-NMR of compound **M5**, Figure S12. FT-IR of compound **M2**, Figure S13. FT-IR of compound **M3**, Figure S14. FT-IR of compound **M4**, Figure S15. FT-IR of compound **M5**, Figure S16. View of independent molecules in the unit cell of **M2** (A) and **M3** (B) with numbering, Figure S17. View of independent molecules in the unit cell of **M5** with numbering, Figure S18. Views of crystal packings of **M2** (A), **M3** (B) and **M5** (C) are shown in the left. Detail view of molecular self-assembly is shown in the right. Independent molecules in the unit cells are colored. H atoms are omitted for clarity, Figure S19. Comparison between 2D fingerprint plots for **M2** (A), **M3** (B) and **M5** (C), Figure S20. Normalized UV-Visible and fluorescence spectra of **M2-M3** and **M5**, Figure S21. DSC of compound **M2** (3 cycles at 10 °C/min), Figure S22. DSC of compound **M3** (3 cycles at 10 °C/min), Figure S23. DSC of compound **M4** (3 cycles at 10 °C/min), Figure S24. DSC of compound **M5** (3 cycles at 10 °C/min), Figure S25. Selected POM images of compound **M2**. Left side: Registered at 132 °C during the cooling cycle (rate 1 °C/min), showing N* phase. Right side: Registered at 119 °C during the cooling cycle (rate 1 °C/min), showing the transition from N* to crystalline phase, Figure S26. Selected POM images of compound **M5**, registered at 204.3 °C during the cooling cycle (rate 0.5 °C/min), showing N* phase from Isotropic, Table S1. Crystal and Structure Refinement data for **M2**, **M3** and **M5**, Table S2. Selected bond lengths for **M2**, **M3** and **M5**, Table S3. Bond lengths for **M2**, **M3** and **M5**, Table S4. Bond angles for **M2**, **M3** and **M5**.

Author Contributions: Manuscript conception, R.N. and I.M.S.; writing and original draft preparation, R.N. and I.M.S.; synthesis and characterization of derivatives **M2–M5**, A.F.-U. and A.G.-C.; photophysical and liquid crystal, A.F.-U. and A.G.-C.; X-ray analysis, J.G.P.; editing, data analysis and interpretation, A.F.-U., A.G.-C., F.T., C.V., R.N. and I.M.S. All authors have read and agreed to the published version of the manuscript.

Funding: This research was funded by MICINN grants (PID2019-106832RB-100 and CEX2019-000917-S) and Generalitat de Catalunya (2017/SGR/1720).

Acknowledgments: This work was supported by Agencia Estatal de Investigación AEI from MICINN (CTQ2016-75150-R and PID2019-106832RB-100/AEI/10.13039/501100011033 project) and Generalitat de Catalunya (2017 SGR1720 projects). The work was also supported by the MICINN through the Severo Ochoa Program for Centers of Excellence FUNFUTURE (CEX2019-000917-S). We gratefully acknowledge A. Whitwood for collecting the X-ray single crystals diffraction pattern.

Conflicts of Interest: The authors declare no conflict of interest. The funders had no role in the design of the study; in the collection, analyses, or interpretation of data; in the writing of the manuscript, or in the decision to publish the results.

References

1. Saez, I.M. Supermolecular Liquid Crystals. In *Handbook of Liquid Crystals*, 2nd ed.; Goodby, J.W., Collings, P.J., Kato, T., Tschierske, C., Gleeson, H., Raynes, P., Vill, V., Eds.; Wiley-VCH: Weinheim, Germany, 2014; Volume 7, pp. 211–258.
2. Saez, I.M. Supermolecular Liquid Crystals. In *Supramolecular Soft Matter*; Nakanishi, T., Ed.; Wiley: Hoboken, NJ, USA, 2011; pp. 301–321.
3. Saez, I.M.; Goodby, J.W. Supermolecular Liquid Crystals. In *Liquid Crystalline Functional Assemblies and Their Supramolecular Structures, Structure and Bonding*; Kato, T., Ed.; Springer: Berlin/Heidelberg, Germany, 2008; Volume 128, pp. 1–62.
4. Wang, Y.; Li, Q. Light-Driven Chiral Molecular Switches or Motors in Liquid Crystals. *Adv. Mater.* **2012**, *24*, 1926. [CrossRef]
5. Mulder, D.J.; Schenning, A.; Bastiaansen, C.W.M. Chiral-nematic liquid crystals as one-dimensional photonic materials in optical sensors. *J. Mater. Chem. C* **2014**, *2*, 6695–6705. [CrossRef]
6. Moirangthem, M.; Arts, R.; Merkx, M.; Schenning, A.P. An optical sensor based on a photonic polymer film to detect calcium in serum. *Adv. Funct. Mater.* **2016**, *26*, 1154–1160. [CrossRef]
7. Ryabchun, A.; Lancia, F.; Chen, J.; Morozov, D.; Feringa, B.L.; Katsonis, N. Helix Inversion Controlled by Molecular Motors in Multistate Liquid Crystals. *Adv. Mater.* **2020**, *32*, 2004420. [CrossRef]
8. Grimes, R.N. *Carboranes*, 3rd ed.; Academic Press: Cambridge, MA, USA, 2016.
9. Issa, F.; Kassiou, M.; Rendina, L.M. Boron in drug discovery: Carboranes as unique pharmacophores in biologically active compounds. *Chem. Rev.* **2011**, *111*, 5701–5722. [CrossRef] [PubMed]
10. Scholz, M.; Hey-Hawkins, E. Carbaboranes as Pharmacophores: Properties, Synthesis, and Application Strategies. *Chem. Rev.* **2011**, *111*, 7035–7062. [CrossRef] [PubMed]
11. Stockmann, P.; Gozzi, M.; Kuhnert, R.; Sárosi, M.B.; Hey-Hawkins, E. New keys for old locks: Carborane-containing drugs as platforms for mechanism-based therapies. *Chem. Soc. Rev.* **2019**, *48*, 3497–3512. [CrossRef] [PubMed]
12. Chen, Z.; King, R.B. Spherical Aromaticity: Recent Work on Fullerenes, Polyhedral Boranes, and Related Structures. *Chem. Rev.* **2005**, *105*, 3613–3642. [CrossRef]
13. Poater, J.; Solà, M.; Viñas, C.; Teixidor, F. A Simple Link between Hydrocarbon and Borohydride Chemistries. *Chem. Eur. J.* **2013**, *19*, 4169–4175. [CrossRef]
14. Poater, J.; Solà, M.; Viñas, C.; Teixidor, F. π-Aromaticity and three-dimensional aromaticity: Two sides of the same coin? *Angew. Chem. Int. Ed.* **2014**, *53*, 12191–12195. [CrossRef]

15. Poater, J.; Sola, M.; Viñas, C.; Teixidor, F. Huckel's Rule of Aromaticity Categorizes Aromatic closo Boron Hydride Clusters. *Chem. Eur. J.* **2016**, *22*, 7437–7443. [CrossRef] [PubMed]
16. Poater, J.; Viñas, C.; Bennour, I.; Escayola, S.; Sola, M.; Teixidor, F. Too Persistent to Give Up: Aromaticity in Boron Clusters Survives Radical Structural Changes. *J. Am. Chem. Soc.* **2020**, *142*, 9396–9407. [CrossRef] [PubMed]
17. Núñez, R.; Farràs, P.; Teixidor, F.; Viñas, C.; Sillanpää, R.; Kivekäs, R. A discrete P···I I···P assembly: The large influence of weak interactions on the ^{31}P NMR Spectra of Phosphane–Diiodine Complexes. *Angew. Chem. Int. Ed.* **2006**, *45*, 1270–1272. [CrossRef] [PubMed]
18. Núñez, R.; Teixidor, F.; Kivekäs, R.; Sillanpää, R.; Viñas, C. Influence of the solvent and R groups on the structure of (carboranyl)R_2PI_2 compounds in solution. Crystal structure of the first iodophosphonium salt incorporating the anion [7,8-nido-C2B9H10]−. *Dalton Trans.* **2008**, 1471–1480.
19. Kolel-Veetil, M.K.; Keller, T.M. Formation of elastomeric network polymers from ambient heterogeneous hydrosilations of carboranylenesiloxane and branched siloxane monomers. *Polym. Sci. Part A* **2006**, *44*, 147–155. [CrossRef]
20. Ferrer-Ugalde, A.; Juárez-Pérez, E.J.; Teixidor, F.; Viñas, C.; Núñez, R. Synthesis, Characterization, and Thermal Behavior of Carboranyl–Styrene Decorated Octasilsesquioxanes: Influence of the Carborane Clusters on Photoluminescence. *Chem. Eur. J.* **2013**, *19*, 17021–17030. [CrossRef]
21. Núñez, R.; Romero, I.; Teixidor, F.; Viñas, C. Icosahedral boron clusters: A perfect tool for the enhancement of polymer features. *Chem. Soc. Rev.* **2016**, *45*, 5147–5173. [CrossRef]
22. Hosmane, N.S. *Boron Science: New Technologies and Applications*; Taylor & Francis: Bosa Roca, USA, 2012.
23. González-Campo, A.; Ferrer-Ugalde, A.; Viñas, C.; Teixidor, F.; Sillanpää, R.; Rodríguez-Romero, J.; Santillan, R.; Farfán, N.; Núñez, R. A Versatile Methodology for the Controlled Synthesis of Photoluminescent High-Boron-Content Dendrimers. *Chem. Eur. J.* **2013**, *19*, 6299–6312. [CrossRef]
24. Hosmane, N.S.; Eagling, R. *Handbook of Boron Chemistry in Organometallics Catalysis, Materials and Medicine*; World Science Publishers: Hackensack, NJ, USA, 2018.
25. Teixidor, F.; Viñas, C.; Demonceau, A.; Nuñez, R. Boron clusters: Do they receive the deserved interest? *Pure Appl. Chem.* **2003**, *75*, 1305–1313. [CrossRef]
26. Lesnikowski, Z.J. Boron units as pharmacophores—New applications and opportunities of boron cluster chemistry. *Collect. Czechoslov. Chem. Commun.* **2007**, *72*, 1646–1658. [CrossRef]
27. Dash, B.P.; Satapathy, R.; Gaillard, E.R.; Norton, K.M.; Maguire, J.A.; Chug, N.; Hosmane, N.S. Enhanced π-conjugation and emission via icosahedral carboranes: Synthetic and spectroscopic investigation. *Inorg. Chem.* **2011**, *50*, 5485–5493. [CrossRef] [PubMed]
28. Weber, L.; Kahlert, J.; Brockhinke, R.; Bohling, L.; Brockhinke, A.; Stammler, H.-G.; Neumann, B.; Harder, R.A.; Fox, M.A. Luminescence properties of C-diazaborolyl-ortho-carboranes as donor-acceptor systems. *Chem. Eur. J.* **2012**, *18*, 8347–8357. [CrossRef] [PubMed]
29. Wee, K.-R.; Cho, Y.-J.; Song, J.K.; Kang, S.O. Multiple photoluminescence from 1,2-dinaphthyl-ortho-carborane. *Angew. Chem. Int. Ed.* **2013**, *52*, 9682–9685. [CrossRef] [PubMed]
30. Guo, J.; Liu, D.; Zhang, J.; Zhang, J.; Miao, Q.; Xie, Z. o-Carborane functionalized pentacenes: Synthesis, molecular packing and ambipolar organic thin-film transistors. *Chem. Commun.* **2015**, *51*, 12004–12007. [CrossRef]
31. Kim, S.-Y.; Lee, A.-R.; Jin, G.F.; Cho, Y.-J.; Son, H.-J.; Han, W.-S.; Kang, S.O. Lectronic Alteration on Oligothiophenes by o-Carborane: Electron Acceptor Character of o-Carborane in Oligothiophene Frameworks with Dicyano-Vinyl End-On Group. *J. Org. Chem.* **2015**, *80*, 4573–4580. [CrossRef] [PubMed]
32. Park, J.; Lee, Y.H.; Ryu, J.Y.; Lee, J.; Lee, M.H. The substituent effect of 2-R-o-carborane on the photophysical properties of iridium(iii) cyclometalates. *Dalton Trans.* **2016**, *45*, 5667–5675. [CrossRef]
33. Tu, D.; Leong, P.; Li, Z.; Hu, R.; Shi, C.; Zhang, K.Y.; Yan, H.; Zhao, Q. A carborane-triggered metastable charge transfer state leading to spontaneous recovery of mechanochromic luminescence. *Chem. Commun.* **2016**, *52*, 12494–12497. [CrossRef]
34. Núñez, R.; Tarrès, M.; Ferrer-Ugalde, A.; de Biani, F.F.; Teixidor, F. Electrochemistry and Photoluminescence of Icosahedral Carboranes, Boranes, Metallacarboranes, and Their Derivatives. *Chem. Rev.* **2016**, *116*, 14307–14378. [CrossRef]
35. Mukherjee, S.; Thilagar, P. Boron clusters in luminescent materials. *Chem. Commun.* **2016**, *52*, 1070–1093. [CrossRef]
36. Naito, H.; Nishino, K.; Morisaki, Y.; Tanaka, K.; Chujo, Y. Solid-State Emission of the Anthracene-o-Carborane Dyad from the Twisted-Intramolecular Charge Transfer in the Crystalline State. *Angew. Chem. Int. Ed.* **2017**, *56*, 254–259. [CrossRef]
37. Wu, X.; Guo, J.; Quan, Y.; Jia, W.; Jia, D.; Chen, Y.; Xie, Z. Cage carbon-substitute does matter for aggregation-induced emission features of o-carborane-functionalized anthracene triads. *J. Mater. Chem. C* **2018**, *6*, 4140–4149. [CrossRef]
38. Nghia, N.V.; Jana, S.; Sujith, S.; Ryu, J.Y.; Lee, J.; Lee, S.U.; Lee, M.H. Nido-Carboranes: Donors for Thermally Activated Delayed Fluorescence. *Angew. Chem. Int. Ed.* **2018**, *57*, 12483–12488. [CrossRef] [PubMed]
39. Martin, K.L.; Smith, J.N.; Young, E.R.; Carter, K.R. Synthetic Emission Tuning of Carborane-Containing Poly(dihexylfluorene)s. *Macromolecules* **2019**, *52*, 7951–7960. [CrossRef]
40. Wei, X.; Zhu, M.-J.; Cheng, Z.; Lee, M.; Yan, H.; Lu, C.; Xu, J.J. Aggregation-Induced Electrochemiluminescence of Carboranyl Carbazoles in Aqueous Media. *Angew. Chem.* **2019**, *131*, 3194–3198. [CrossRef]
41. Ochi, J.; Tanaka, K.; Chujo, Y. Recent Progress in the Development of Solid-State Luminescent o-Carboranes with Stimuli Responsivity. *Angew. Chem. Int. Ed.* **2020**, *59*, 9841–9855. [CrossRef]

42. Ferrer-Ugalde, A.; Juárez-Pérez, E.J.; Teixidor, F.; Viñas, C.; Sillanpää, R.; Pérez Inestrosa, E.; Núñez, R. Synthesis and Characterization of New Fluorescent Styrene Containing Carborane Derivatives. The singular quenching role of a Phenyl Substituent. *Chem. Eur. J.* **2012**, *18*, 544–553. [CrossRef]
43. Ferrer-Ugalde, A.; González-Campo, A.; Viñas, C.; Rodríguez-Romero, J.; Santillan, R.; Farfán, N.; Sillanpää, R.; Sousa-Pedrares, A.; Núñez, R.; Teixidor, F. Fluorescence of New o-Carborane Compounds with Different Fluorophores: Can It Be Tuned? *Chem. Eur. J.* **2014**, *20*, 9940–9951. [CrossRef]
44. Cabrera-González, J.; Viñas, C.; Haukka, M.; Bhattacharyya, S.; Gierschner, J.; Núñez, R. Photoluminescence in Carborane-Stilbene Triads: A Structural, Spectroscopic, and Computational Study. *Chem. Eur. J.* **2016**, *22*, 13588–13598. [CrossRef]
45. Cabrera-González, J.; Bhattacharyya, S.; Milián-Medina, B.; Teixidor, F.; Farfán, N.; Arcos-Ramos, R.; Vargas-Reyes, V.; Gierschner, J.; Núñez, R. Tetrakis{[(p-dodecacarboranyl)methyl]stilbenyl}ethylene: A Luminescent Tetraphenylethylene (TPE) Core System. *Eur. J. Inorg. Chem.* **2017**, 4575–4580. [CrossRef]
46. Ferrer-Ugalde, A.; Cabrera-González, J.; Juárez-Pérez, E.J.; Teixidor, F.; Pérez-Inestrosa, E.; Montenegro, J.M.; Sillanpää, R.; Haukka, M.; Núñez, R. Carborane–stilbene dyads: The influence of substituents and cluster isomers on photoluminescence properties. *Dalton Trans.* **2017**, *46*, 2091–2104. [CrossRef] [PubMed]
47. Cabrera-González, J.; Ferrer-Ugalde, A.; Bhattacharyya, S.; Chaari, M.; Teixidor, F.; Gierschner, J.; Núñez, R. Fluorescent carborane–vinylstilbene functionalised octasilsesquioxanes: Synthesis, structural, thermal and photophysical properties. *J. Mater. Chem. C* **2017**, *5*, 10211–10219. [CrossRef]
48. Bellomo, C.; Chaari, M.; Cabrera-González, J.; Blangetti, M.; Lombardi, C.; Deagostino, A.; Viñas, C.; Gaztelumendi, N.; Nogués, C.; Nuñez, R.; et al. Carborane-BODIPY Dyads: New Photoluminescent Materials through an Efficient Heck Coupling. *Chem. Eur. J.* **2018**, *24*, 15622–15630. [CrossRef] [PubMed]
49. Li, X.-Q.; Wang, C.-H.; Zhang, M.-Y.; Zou, H.-Y.; Ma, N.-N.; Qiu, Y.-Q. Tuning second-order nonlinear optical properties of the two-dimensional benzene/carborane compounds with phenyl carbazoles: Substituent effect and redox switch. *J. Organomet. Chem.* **2014**, *749*, 327–334. [CrossRef]
50. Wang, J.; Wang, W.-Y.; Fang, X.-Y.; Qiu, Y.-Q. Carborane tuning on iridium complexes: Redox-switchable second-order NLO responses. *J. Mol. Model.* **2015**, *21*, 95. [CrossRef]
51. Kaszynski, P. *Boron Science: New Technologies and Applications*; Hosmane, N.S., Ed., CRC Press & Taylor and Frances Group: Boca Raton, FL, USA, 2012; p. 319.
52. Nagamine, T.; Januszko, A.; Ohta, K.; Kaszynski, P.; Endo, Y. The effect of the linking group on mesogenic properties of three-ring derivatives of p-carborane and biphenyl. *Liq. Cryst.* **2008**, *35*, 865–884. [CrossRef]
53. Piecek, W.; Glab, K.L.; Januszko, A.; Perkowski, P.; Kaszynski, P. Modification of electro-optical properties of an orthoconic chiral biphenyl smectogen with its isostructural carborane analogue. *J. Mater. Chem.* **2009**, *19*, 1173–1182. [CrossRef]
54. Ringstrand, B.; Jankowiak, A.; Johnson, L.E.; Kaszynski, P.; Pociechacand, D.; Górecka, E. Anion-driven mesogenicity: A comparative study of ionic liquid crystals basedon the [closo-1-CB9H10]- and [closo-1-CB11H12]- clusters. *J. Mater. Chem.* **2012**, *22*, 4874–4880. [CrossRef]
55. Pecyna, J.; Pociecha, D.; Kaszynski, P. Zwitterionic pyridinium derivatives of [closo-1-CB9H10]- and [closo-1-CB11H12]- clusters as as high De additives to a nematic host. *J. Mater. Chem. C* **2014**, *2*, 1585–1591. [CrossRef]
56. Fisher, S.P.; Tomich, A.W.; Lovera, S.O.; Kleinsasser, J.F.; Guo, J.; Asay, M.J.; Nelson, H.M.; Lavallo, V. Nonclassical Applications of closo-Carborane Anions: From Main Group Chemistry and Catalysis to Energy Storage. *Chem. Rev.* **2019**, *119*, 8262–8290. [CrossRef] [PubMed]
57. Ali, M.O.; Lasseter, J.C.; Żurawiński, R.; Pietrzak, A.; Pecyna, J.; Wojciechowski, J.; Friedli, A.C.; Pociecha, D.; Kaszyński, P. Thermal and Photophysical Properties of Highly Quadrupolar Liquid-Crystalline Derivatives of the [closo-B12H12](2-) Anion. *Chem. Eur. J.* **2019**, *25*, 2616–2630. [CrossRef]
58. Ringstrand, B.; Kaszynski, P. Investigation of high $\Delta\varepsilon$ derivatives of the [closo-1-CB9H10]- anion for liquid crystal display applications. *J. Mat. Chem.* **2011**, *21*, 90–95. [CrossRef]
59. Pecyna, J.; Denicola, R.P.; Gray, H.M.; Ringstrand, B.; Kaszynski, P. The effect of molecular polarity on nem/catic phase stability in 12-vertex carboranes. *Liq. Cryst.* **2014**, *41*, 1188–1198. [CrossRef]
60. Januszko, A.; Glab, K.L.; Kaszynski, P. Induction of smectic behaviour in a carborane-containing mesogen. Tail fluorination of a threering nematogen and its miscibility with benzene analogues. *Liq. Cryst.* **2008**, *35*, 549. [CrossRef]
61. Feakes, D.A.; Spinler, J.K.; Harris, F.R. Synthesis of boron-containing cholesterol derivatives for incorporation into unilamellar liposomes and evaluation as potential agents for BNCT. *Tetrahedron* **1999**, *55*, 11177–11186. [CrossRef]
62. Nakamura, H.; Miyajima, Y.; Takei, T.; Kasaoka, S.; Maruyama, K. Synthesis and vesicle formation of a nido-carborane cluster lipid for boron neutron capture therapy. *Chem. Commun.* **2004**, 1910–1911. [CrossRef] [PubMed]
63. Feakes, D.A.; Shelly, K.; Hawthorne, M.F. Selective boron delivery to murine tumors by lipophilic species incorporated in the membranes of unilamellar liposomes. *Proc. Natl. Acad. Sci. USA* **1995**, *92*, 1367–1370. [CrossRef] [PubMed]
64. Bregadze, V.I.; Sivaev, I.B.; Dubey, R.D.; Semioshkin, A.; Shmal'ko, A.V.; Kosenko, I.D.; Lebedeva, K.V.; Mandal, S.; Sreejyothi, P.; Sarkar, A.; et al. Boron-Containing Lipids and Liposomes: New Conjugates of Cholesterol with Polyhedral Boron Hydrides. *Chem. Eur. J.* **2020**, *20*, 13832–13841. [CrossRef] [PubMed]
65. Jankowiak, A.; Kaszynski, P. Practical Synthesis of 1,12-Difunctionalized o-Carborane for the Investigation of Polar Liquid Crystals. *Inorg. Chem.* **2014**, *53*, 8762–8769. [CrossRef] [PubMed]

66. Pecyna, J.; Jankowiak, A.; Pociecha, D.; Kaszyński, P. o-Carborane derivatives for probing molecular polarity effects on liquid crystal phase stability and dielectric behavior. *J. Mater. Chem. C.* **2015**, *3*, 11412–11422. [CrossRef]
67. Saez, I.M.; Goodby, J.W. Chiral nematic octasilsesquioxanes. *J. Mater. Chem.* **2001**, *11*, 2845–2855. [CrossRef]
68. Saez, I.M.; Goodby, J.W.; Richardson, R.M. A liquid-crystalline silsesquioxane dendrimer exhibiting chiral nematic and columnar mesophases. *Chem. Eur. J.* **2001**, 2758–2764. [CrossRef]
69. Felder-Flesch, D.; Rupnicki, L.; Bourgogne, C.; Donnio, B.; Guillon, D. Liquid-crystalline cholesterol-based [60]fullerene hexaadducts. *J. Mater. Chem.* **2006**, *16*, 304–309. [CrossRef]
70. Campidelli, S.; Brandmüller, T.; Hirsch, A.; Saez, I.M.; Goodby, J.W.; Deschenaux, R. An Optically-active Liquid-crystalline Hexa-adduct of [60]Fullerene which Displays Supramolecular Helical Organization. *Chem. Comm.* **2006**, *41*, 4282–4284. [CrossRef] [PubMed]
71. Campidelli, S.; Bourgun, P.; Guintchin, B.; Furrer, J.; Stoeckli-Evans, H.; Saez, I.M.; Goodby, J.W.; Deschenaux, R. Diastereoisomerically Pure Fulleropyrrolidines as Chiral Platforms for the Design of Optically Active Liquid Crystals. *J. Am. Chem. Soc.* **2010**, *132*, 3574–3581. [CrossRef]
72. Gresham, K.D.; McHugh, C.M.; Bunning, T.J.; Crane, R.L.; Klei, H.E.; Samulski, E.T. Phase behavior of cyclic siloxane-based liquid crystalline compounds. *J. Polym. Sci. Part A Polym. Chem.* **1994**, *32*, 2039–2047. [CrossRef]
73. Trinh, T.M.N.; Nguyen, T.T.; Kopp, C.; Pieper, P.; Ruso, V.; Heinrich, B.; Donnio, B.; Nguyen, T.L.A.; Deschenaux, R. Olefin Cross-Metathesis: A Versatile Synthetic Reaction for the Design of Janus Liquid Crystals. *Eur. J. Org. Chem.* **2015**, *27*, 6005–6010. [CrossRef]
74. Russo, V.; Pieper, P.; Heinrich, B.; Donnio, B.; Deschenaux, R. Design, Synthesis, and Self-Assembly Behavior of Liquid Crystalline Bis-[60]Fullerodendrimers. *Chem. Eur. J.* **2016**, *22*, 17366–17376. [CrossRef]
75. Zep, A.; Pruszkowska, K.; Dobrzycki, Ł.; Sektas, K.; Szałański, P.; Marek, P.H.; Cyrański, M.K.; Sicinski, R.R. Cholesterol-based photo-switchable mesogenic dimers. Strongly bent molecules versus an intercalated structure. *CrystEngComm* **2019**, *21*, 2779–2789. [CrossRef]
76. Fox, M.A.; Hughes, A.K. Cage C-H···X interactions in solid-state structures of icosahedral carboranes. *Coord. Chem. Rev.* **2004**, *248*, 457–476. [CrossRef]
77. Turn, M.J.; McKinnon, J.J.; Wolff, S.K.; Grimwood, D.J.; Spackman, P.R.; Jayatilaka, D.; Spackman, M.A. CrystalExplorer17. University of Western Australia, 2017. Available online: https://crystalexplorer.scb.uwa.edu.au (accessed on 27 January 2021).
78. Di Salvo, F.; Camargo, B.; Garcia, Y.; Teixidor, F.; Viñas, C.; Giner Planas, J.; Light, M.E.; Hursthouse, M.B. Supramolecular architectures in o-carboranyl alcohols bearing N-aromatic rings: Syntheses, crystal structures and melting points correlation. *CrystEngComm* **2011**, *13*, 5788–5806. [CrossRef]
79. Dierking, I. *Textures of Liquid Crystals*; Wiley-VCH Verlag GmbH & Co. KGaA: Weinheim, Germany, 2003.
80. Cowling, S.J.; Hall, A.W.; Goodby, J.W. Effect of terminal functional group size on ferroelectric and antiferroelectric properties of liquid crystals. *Liq. Cryst.* **2005**, *32*, 1483–1498. [CrossRef]
81. Oxford Diffraction Ltd. *CrysAlisPro. Version 1.171.34.40 (Release 27–08-2010 CrysAlis171. NET) (Compiled 27 August 2010, 11:50:40) Empirical Absorption Correction using Spherical Harmonics, Implemented in SCALE3 ABSPACK Scaling Algorithm*; Oxford Diffraction Ltd.: Abingdon, UK, 2010.
82. Sheldrick, G.M. A short history of SHELX. *Acta Cryst.* **2008**, *A64*, 112–122. [CrossRef] [PubMed]
83. Palatinus, L.; Chapuis, G. SUPERFLIP—A computer program for the solution of crystal structures by charge flipping in arbitrary dimensions. *J. Appl. Cryst.* **2007**, *40*, 786–790. [CrossRef]
84. Dolomanov, O.V.; Bourhis, L.J.; Gildea, R.J.; Howard, J.A.; Puschmann, H. OLEX2: A complete structure solution, refinement and analysis program. *J. Appl. Crystallogr.* **2009**, *42*, 339–341. [CrossRef]

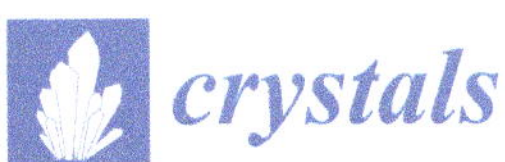 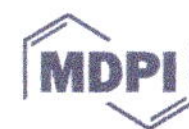

Article

Exploration of Bis(nickelation) of 1,1′-Bis(*o*-carborane)

Dipendu Mandal *,† and Georgina M. Rosair *

Institute of Chemical Sciences, School of Engineering & Physical Sciences, Heriot-Watt University, Edinburgh EH14 4AS, UK
* Correspondence: chmdip@nus.edu.sg (D.M.); g.m.rosair@hw.ac.uk (G.M.R.)
† Present address: Department of Chemistry, National University of Singapore, 3 Science Drive 3, Singapore 117543, Singapore.

Abstract: The metalation of $[Tl]_2[1\text{-}(1'\text{-}3',1',2'\text{-}closo\text{-}TlC_2B_9H_{10})\text{-}3,1,2\text{-}closo\text{-}TlC_2B_9H_{10}]$, with the smaller {Ni(dmpe)} fragment sourced from $[Ni(dmpe)Cl_2]$, is explored. The bis(metalated) products are obtained as a diastereoisomeric mixture. These isomers were separated, fully characterised spectroscopically and crystallographically and identified as *rac*-$[1\text{-}(1'\text{-}3'\text{-}(dmpe)\text{-}3',1',2'\text{-}closo\text{-}NiC_2B_9H_{10})\text{-}3\text{-}(dmpe)\text{-}3,1,2\text{-}closo\text{-}NiC_2B_9H_{10}]$ (**1**) and *meso*-$[1\text{-}(1'\text{-}3'\text{-}(dmpe)\text{-}3',1',2'\text{-}closo\text{-}NiC_2B_9H_{10})\text{-}3\text{-}(dmpe)\text{-}3,1,2\text{-}closo\text{-}NiC_2B_9H_{10}]$ (**2**). Previously, these $3,1,2\text{-}NiC_2B_9\text{-}3',1',2'\text{-}NiC_2B_9$ architectures (where both cages are not isomerised), were inaccessible, and thus new structures can be achieved during bis(nickelation) with {Ni(dmpe)}. Further, the metalation of the tetra-thallium salt with the bulky {Ni(dppe)} fragment sourced from $[Ni(dppe)Cl_2]$ was also studied. These bis(nickelated) products were also fully characterised and are afforded as the stereospecific species *rac*-$[1\text{-}(1'\text{-}3'\text{-}(dppe)\text{-}3',1',2'\text{-}closo\text{-}NiC_2B_9H_{10})\text{-}3\text{-}(dppe)\text{-}3,1,2\text{-}closo\text{-}NiC_2B_9H_{10}]$ (**3**) and $[1\text{-}(2'\text{-}4'\text{-}(dppe)\text{-}4',1',2'\text{-}closo\text{-}NiC_2B_9H_{10})\text{-}3\text{-}(dppe)\text{-}3,1,2\text{-}closo\text{-}NiC_2B_9H_{10}]$ (**4**α). In the latter metalation, compound **3** shows intramolecular dihydrogen bonding, contributing to the stereospecificity, whereas isomerisation from 3,1,2 to 4,1,2- in the **4**α is related to steric relief.

Keywords: 1,1′-bis(*o*-carborane); deboronation; metalation; bis(nickelation); diastereoisomers; stereospecific

Citation: Mandal, D.; Rosair, G.M. Exploration of Bis(nickelation) of 1,1′-Bis(*o*-carborane). *Crystals* **2021**, *11*, 16. https://dx.doi.org/10.3390/cryst11010016

Received: 10 December 2020
Accepted: 22 December 2020
Published: 27 December 2020

1. Introduction

Since the discovery of bis(carboranes) in 1964, the chemistry of 1,1′-bis(*o*-carborane) (Scheme 1, **a**) has evolved rapidly, particularly once a high-yielding synthetic route was devised in 2003. Bis(carborane) offers a versatile building block in designing three-dimensional molecules, an array of homogeneous catalyst precursors, luminescent materials and organic derivatives via C_{cage}-H or B_{cage}-H functionalisation [1–6].

Since 2010, the Welch group have established many variations of the metalation chemistry of 1,1′-bis(*o*-carborane), one approach being cage expansion chemistry via reduction-metalation of this species [1], whilst another metalation strategy explored broadly within the group is deboronation/metalation of 1,1′-bis(*o*-carborane).

The single deboronation/metalation of 1,1′-bis(*o*-carborane) has been reported for cobalt, nickel and ruthenium metal fragments and afforded a wide range of mono-metallic-bis(carborane) isomers [7,8]. In further developments, double deboronation/metalation was achieved, such that both cages became metallacarboranes. The bimetallic metallacarboranes derived from the metalation of doubly deboronated 1,1′-bis(*o*-carborane) with both rhodium and ruthenium fragments are $3,1,2\text{-}MC_2B_9\text{-}2',1',8'\text{-}MC_2B_9$ [M = {Rh}, {Ru}] species, in which one of the cages has isomerised (Scheme 1, **b** and **c**). There are limited examples of the parent $3,1,2\text{-}MC_2B_9\text{-}3',1',2'\text{-}MC_2B_9$ form [9,10]. Variation in the isomer type with cobalt has been achieved by varying the metalation source, forming either $3,1,2\text{-}CoC_2B_9\text{-}3',1',2'\text{-}CoC_2B_9$ (non-isomerised) or $3,1,2\text{-}CoC_2B_9\text{-}2',1',8'\text{-}CoC_2B_9$ (isomerised) (Scheme 1, **c**) products [9]. Notably, an example of stepwise deboronation/metalation-deboronation/heterometalation is also reported [11]. Here we document an expansion of the bimetallic metallacarboranes library via the double deboronation/nickelation of 1,1′-bis(*o*-carborane).

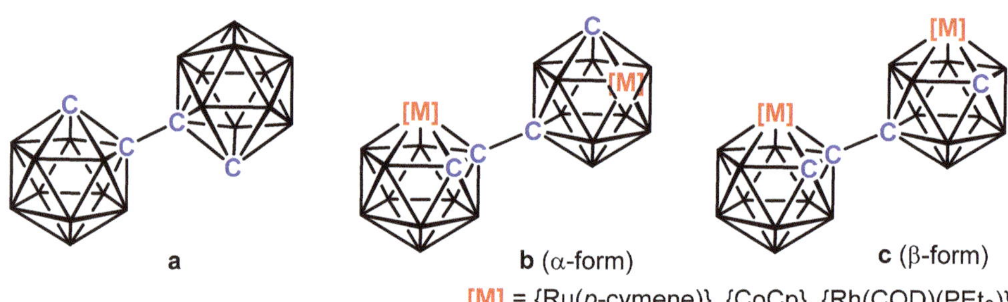

Scheme 1. Line diagrams of **a**–**c**. Species **a** is 1,1′-bis(*o*-carborane), whereas **b** (α-form) and **c** (β-form) were derived via double deboronation/metalation of **a**. Unlabelled vertices are B.

2. Materials and Methods

2.1. General Considerations

Experiments were carried out under dry, oxygen-free N_2, using standard Schlenk techniques, although subsequent manipulations were performed at ambient condition. Tetrahydrofuran (THF) was dried and distilled under sodium/benzophenone, whilst petrol was distilled from sodium wire before use. DCM was purified in an MBRAUN SPS-800(Dieselstr. 31, D-85748 Garching,). Degassing of solvents was performed (3 × freeze-pump-thaw cycles) before reaction. Preparative TLC used Kieselgel F_{254} glass plates (20 × 20 cm). ^{1}H (400.1 MHz), ^{31}P (162.0 MHz) or ^{11}B (128.4 MHz) NMR spectra and ^{1}H-^{31}P Heteronuclear Multiple Bond Correlation (HMBC) experiment (in Supplementary Materials) were run on a Bruker DPX-400 spectrometer (Bruker BioSpin AG, Fallenden, Switzerland). The precursors 1,1′-bis(*o*-carborane) [12], its deboronated derivative $[Tl]_2$[1-(1′-3′,1′,2′-*closo*-$TlC_2B_9H_{10}$)-3,1,2-*closo*-$TlC_2B_9H_{10}$] (Tl_4-salt) (WARNING: Thallium is extremely toxic, appropriate precautions are required when handling thallium compounds) [9] and [$NiCl_2$ (dmpe)] (dmpe = 1,2-bis(dimethylphosphino)ethane) [13] were prepared by modified literature methods. [$NiCl_2$(dppe)] (dppe = 1,2-bis(diphenylphosphino)ethane) and the remaining reagents were purchased commercially.

2.1.1. Synthesis and Characterisation of *rac*-[1-(1′-3′-(dmpe)-3′,1′,2′-*closo*-$NiC_2B_9H_{10}$)-3-(dmpe)-3,1,2-*closo*-$NiC_2B_9H_{10}$] (**1**) and *meso*-[1-(1′-3′-(dmpe)-3′,1′,2′-*closo*-$NiC_2B_9H_{10}$)-3-(dmpe)-3,1,2-*closo*-$NiC_2B_9H_{10}$] (**2**)

The Tl_4-salt (0.60 g, 0.56 mmol) was taken into THF (15 mL). The yellow suspension was degassed by freeze-pump-thaw (three cycles). [$NiCl_2$(dmpe)] (0.31 g, 1.1 mmol) was transferred at −196 °C. The reaction suspension was allowed to warm and was stirred at room temperature. After overnight stirring, the mixture turned dark green. All volatiles were removed *in vacuo*. The residue was dissolved in DCM and passed through a small pad of silica. The filtrate was reduced in volume under low pressure and purified by preparative TLC using DCM and petrol (80:20) to afford two dark green bands, which were collected as solids. The upper green band with R_f = 0.84 afforded *rac*-[1-(1′-3′-(dmpe)-3′,1′,2′-*closo*-$NiC_2B_9H_{10}$)-3-(dmpe)-3,1,2-*closo*-$NiC_2B_9H_{10}$] (**1**) (80 mg, 21%) and a lower green band with R_f = 0.63 gave *meso*-[1-(1′-3′-(dmpe)-3′,1′,2′-*closo*-$NiC_2B_9H_{10}$)-3-(dmpe)-3,1,2-*closo*-$NiC_2B_9H_{10}$] (**2**) (76 mg, 20%).

Compound **1**: ^{1}H NMR (CD_2Cl_2): δ 2.43 (d, $^{3}J_{PH}$ = 14.0 Hz, 2H, CH_{cage}), 2.14–1.90 (m, 8H, P{CH_2}$_2$P), 1.83 (d, $^{2}J_{PH}$ = 10.0 Hz, 6H, CH_3), 1.67 (d, $^{2}J_{PH}$ = 10.0 Hz, 6H, CH_3), 1.55 (d, $^{2}J_{PH}$ = 10.0 Hz, 12H, CH_3). ^{1}H{^{31}P} NMR (CD_2Cl_2): δ 2.43 (s, 2H, CH_{cage}), 2.12–1.89 (m, 8H, P{CH_2}$_2$P), 1.83 (s, 6H, CH_3), 1.67 (s, 6H, CH_3), 1.56 (s, 12H, CH_3). ^{31}P{^{1}H} NMR

(CD_2Cl_2): δ 43.1 (d, $^2J_{PP}$ = 29.2 Hz, 2P), 33.0 (d, $^2J_{PP}$ = 29.2 Hz, 2P). $^{11}B\{^1H\}$ NMR (CD_2Cl_2): δ −2.7 (2B), −4.1 (2B), −7.3 (2B), −11.8 (2B), −13.6 (2B), −15.8 (4B), −21.1 (4B).

Compound **2**: ^1H NMR (CD_2Cl_2): δ 2.48 (d, $^3J_{PH}$ = 10.0 Hz, 2H, CH_{cage}), 2.16–1.79 (m, 8H, $P\{CH_2\}_2P$), 1.73 (d, $^2J_{PH}$ = 10.0 Hz, 6H, CH_3), 1.70 (d, $^2J_{PH}$ = 8.0 Hz, 6H, CH_3), 1.57 (d, $^2J_{PH}$ = 10.0 Hz, 6H, CH_3), 1.55 (d, $^2J_{PH}$ = 8.0 Hz, 6H, CH_3). $^1H\{^{31}P\}$ NMR (CD_2Cl_2): δ 2.49 (s, 2H, CH_{cage}), 2.14–1.78 (m, 8H, $P\{CH_2\}_2P$), 1.74 (s, 6H, CH_3), 1.70 (s, 6H, CH_3), 1.57 (s, 6H, CH_3), 1.55 (s, 6H, CH_3). $^{31}P\{^1H\}$ NMR (CD_2Cl_2): δ 43.7 (d, $^2J_{PP}$ = 28.4 Hz, 2P), 33.4 (d, $^2J_{PP}$ = 28.4 Hz, 2P). $^{11}B\{^1H\}$ NMR (CD_2Cl_2): δ−1.5 (2B), −4.0 (2B), −10.4 (2B), −11.5 (2B), −14.5 (3B), −15.9 (5B), −20.4 (2B).

2.1.2. Synthesis and Characterisation of *rac*-[1-(1′-3′-(dppe)-3′,1′,2′-*closo*-$NiC_2B_9H_{10}$)-3-(dppe)-3,1,2-*closo*-$NiC_2B_9H_{10}$] (**3**) and [1-(2′-4′-(dppe)-4′,1′,2′-*closo*–$NiC_2B_9H_{10}$)-3-(dppe)-3,1,2-*closo*-$NiC_2B_9H_{10}$] (**4**α)

A yellow suspension of Tl_4-salt (0.60 g, 0.56 mmol) in THF (20 mL) was frozen at −196 °C. [$NiCl_2$(dppe)] (0.59 g, 1.1 mmol) added to the frozen mixture. After overnight stirring, the reaction mixture gave a green suspension. All volatiles were evaporated off under reduced pressure. The mixture was taken into DCM and filtered through silica. The filtrate was reduced in a minimum amount under low pressure. The mixture was purified by preparative TLC with DCM and petrol (60:40). This yielded, along with a trace amount of purple band with R_f = 0.39, two major mobile components. The lower army-green band with R_f = 0.28 collected as a solid, and after crystallisations, yielded *rac*-[1-(1′-3′-(dppe)-3′,1′,2′-*closo*-$NiC_2B_9H_{10}$)-3-(dppe)-3,1,2-*closo*-$NiC_2B_9H_{10}$] (**3**) (130 mg, 20%). The upper army green-band with R_f = 0.35 afforded [1-(2′-4′-(dppe)-4′,1′,2′-*closo*-$NiC_2B_9H_{10}$)-3-(dppe)-3,1,2-*closo*-$NiC_2B_9H_{10}$] (**4**α) (122 mg, 19%).

Compound **3**: ^1H NMR (CD_2Cl_2): δ 7.80–7.25 (m, 40H, C_6H_5), 3.29–1.96 (m, 8H, $P\{CH_2\}_2P$), 1.83 (d, $^3J_{PH}$ = 11.6 Hz, 2H, CH_{cage}). $^1H\{^{31}P\}$ NMR (CD_2Cl_2): δ 7.79–7.25 (m, 40H, C_6H_5), 3.29–1.97 (m, 8H, $P\{CH_2\}_2P$), 1.84 (s, 2H, CH_{cage}). $^{31}P\{^1H\}$ NMR (CD_2Cl_2): δ 51.6 (d, $^2J_{PP}$ = 19.9 Hz, 2P), 39.2 (d, $^2J_{PP}$ = 19.9 Hz, 2P). $^{11}B\{^1H\}$ NMR (CD_2Cl_2): δ 4.9 (2B), −2.5 (4B), −9.0 (2B), −14.7 (5B), −18.0 (5B).

Compound **4**α: ^1H NMR (CD_2Cl_2): δ 8.01–7.02 (m, 40H, C_6H_5), 3.67–2.26 (m, 8H, $P\{CH_2\}_2P$), 1.94 (s, 1H, CH_{cage}), 1.66 (d, $^3J_{PH}$ = 11.2 Hz, 1H, CH_{cage}). $^1H\{^{31}P\}$ NMR (CD_2Cl_2): δ 8.02–7.01 (m, 40H, C_6H_5), 3.68–2.25 (m, 8H, $P\{CH_2\}_2P$), 1.95 (s, 1H, CH_{cage}), 1.67 (s, 1H, CH_{cage}). $^{31}P\{^1H\}$ NMR (CD_2Cl_2): δ 62.9 (s, 2P), 49.4 (d, $^2J_{PP}$ = 16.6 Hz, 1P), 47.5 (d, $^2J_{PP}$ = 16.6 Hz, 1P). $^{11}B\{^1H\}$ NMR (CD_2Cl_2): δ 5.9 (1B), 1.7 (1B), −0.2 (1B), −4.6 (3B), −9.8 to −20.4 multiple overlapping resonances with maxima at −9.8, −13.5, −15.6, −16.8, −20.4 (total integral of last five resonances 12B).

2.2. *Crystallographic Studies*

X-ray diffraction quality crystals of **1**–**4**α were obtained by solvent diffusion at 5 °C using DCM and petrol 40–60 as antisolvent. Intensity data for compounds **1**–**3** were collected on a Bruker X8 APEXII diffractometer, whereas for compound **4**α on a Rigaku FRE+ equipped with VHF Varimax confocal mirrors and an AFC10 goniometer and HG Saturn 724+ detector using Mo-K_α X-radiation at the UK National Crystallography Service. All crystals were mounted in inert oil on a cryoloop and cooled to 100 K by an Oxford Cryosystems Cryostream. Indexing, data collection and absorption correction were performed using the APEXII suite of programmes [14]. Structures were solved with the SHELXS programme [15] and refined by full-matrix least-squares (SHELXL), using OLEX2 [16]. Table 1 summarises the crystallographic parameters. The location of the CH vertices in all cases was established by the Vertex to Centroid (VCD) method developed by the Welch group [17]. The VCD method is based on the fact that, in a carborane cage, the C vertices are closer to the cage centroid than the B vertices. The CH vertex's location was corroborated by the Boron-to-Hydrogen distance method ("B"–H bond lengths for actual C atoms refined to ca. <0.8Å) in all cases except **4**α, where the positions of the H atoms could not be freely refined against the weak and twinned diffraction data. In this case, B-H distances were restrained to 1.10(2) Å.

Table 1. Crystallographic data for compounds **1–4α**.

	1	**2**	**3**	**4α**
Formula	$C_{16}H_{52}B_{18}Ni_2P_4$	$C_{19}H_{58}B_{18}Cl_6Ni_2P_4$	$C_{59}H_{74}B_{18}Cl_6Ni_2P_4$	$C_{59}H_{74}B_{18}Ni_2P_4Cl_6$
M	680.45	935.23	1431.76	1431.76
Crystal system	monoclinic	triclinic	monoclinic	orthorhombic
Space group	$P2/n$	P-1	C2/c	$P2_12_12_1$
a/Å	13.6195(9)	11.4867(6)	25.0952(8)	10.2816(4)
b/Å	8.7239(5)	12.5327(6)	14.9165(5)	20.3356(9)
c/Å	14.3241(9)	15.0938(8)	19.7053(6)	32.3413(14)
$\alpha/°$	90	96.986(3)	90	90
$\beta/°$	100.316(3)	90.037(3)	113.620(2)	90
$\gamma/°$	90	91.277(2)	90	90
$U/Å^3$	1674.41(18)	2156.21(19)	6758.4(4)	6762.0(5)
Z	2	2	4	4
$D_{calc}g/cm^3$	1.350	1.440	1.407	1.406
μ(Mo-Kα)/mm $^{-1}$	1.328	1.412	0.929	0.928
F(000)/e	708	960	2944	2944
2Θ range/°	5.572 to 52.748	4.462 to 52.206	5.584 to 58.27	4.2 to 55.12
Data measured	46,391	29,045	59,135	45,269
Unique data, n	3479	8280	8989	15,482
Variables	216	520	445	792
S (all data)	1.053	1.031	1.015	0.946
R_{int}	0.0436	0.0517	0.0510	0.1211
R, wR_2 [all data]	0.0258, 0.0498	0.0752, 0.0996	0.0598, 0.0974	0.1200, 0.1892
E_{max}, E_{min}/e $Å^{-3}$	0.29/−0.26	0.87/−0.79	0.65/−1.01	0.52/−0.72
Flack parameter	-	-	-	0.12(2)

1 was treated as a two-component crystal and refined with hklf 5 data. In **4α**, disordered phenyl carbon atoms were constrained to have equal displacement parameters. The crystal of **4α** was not single and refined as a two-component twin with the twin law 1 0 0 0 –1 0 0 0 –1 against HKLF 4 data, which were themselves treated with the solvent mask procedure implemented in OLEX2. HKLF 5 data were not available from the National crystallography service for this structure. A refinement model of the solvent showed approximately three molecules of highly disordered CH_2Cl_2 per bis carborane.

3. Results and Discussion

3.1. Characterisation of Compounds 1 and 2

Previously, the double deboronated [7-(7′-7′,8′-*nido*-$C_2B_9H_{10}$)-7,8-*nido*-$C_2B_9H_{10}$]$^{4-}$ tetraanion derived from [1-(1′-1′,2′-*closo*-$C_2B_{10}H_{11}$)-1,2-*closo*-$C_2B_{10}H_{11}$], commonly called 1,1′-bis(*o*-carborane), was isolated as $[HNMe_3]^+$ or $[BTMA]^+$ [BTMA = benzyltrimethylammonium] salts. Later, $[Tl]^+$ salts were chosen for metalation because of their generally better yields [9]. We have reacted a suspension of $[Tl]_2$[1-(1′-3′,1′,2′-*closo*-$TlC_2B_9H_{10}$)-3,1,2-*closo*-$TlC_2B_9H_{10}$] in THF with [Ni(dmpe)Cl_2] at room temperature. Workup and purification of the dark-green suspension involving preparative thin-layer chromatography (TLC) resulted in two dark green bands, compounds **1** and **2**, in moderate yield (Scheme 2). These were fully characterised by a variety of spectroscopic and crystallographic analyses.

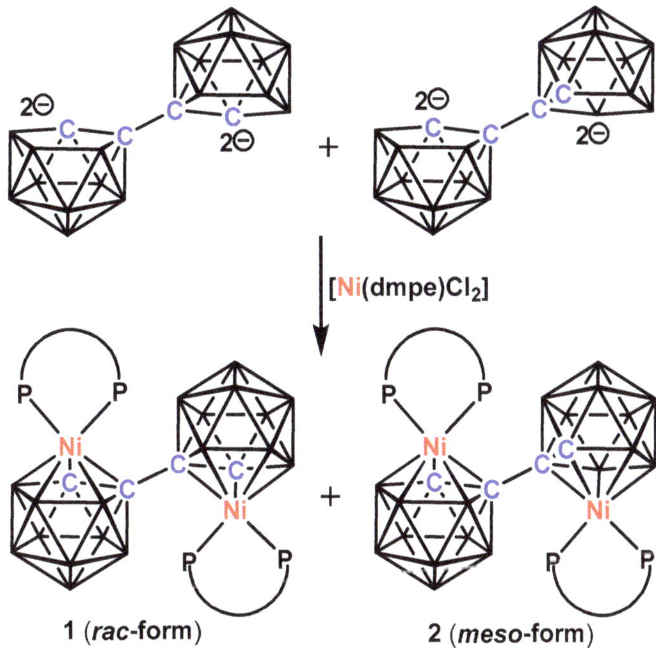

Scheme 2. Synthesis of **1** and **2** from the nickelation of $[Tl]_2[1\text{-}(1'\text{-}3',1',2'\text{-}closo\text{-}TlC_2B_9H_{10})\text{-}3,1,2\text{-}closo\text{-}TlC_2B_9H_{10}]$. NiPP = {Ni(dmpe)}.

An interesting feature of the double deboronation-metalation of 1,1′-bis(*o*-carborane) is that it gives diastereomeric metallcarborane products. Indeed, compound **1** turns out to be *racemic*, whilst compound **2** is in the *meso* form. These observations are also consistent with the NMR spectroscopic analysis. The ^{1}H NMR spectrum of compound **1** reveals resonances arising from the methylene bridge of the two dmpe ligands, whilst the methyl groups of the dmpe ligands produce three doublet resonances. The first two are of integral-6 at δ 1.83, 1.67 ppm with coupling $^2J_{PH}$ = 10.0 Hz, and the last one is of integral-12 at δ 1.55, $^2J_{PH}$ = 10.0 Hz. On the contrary, the ^{1}H NMR spectrum of compound **2** reveals, in addition to the signals for methylene bridge of the dmpe ligands, four doublets assigned to the methyl protons of the dmpe fragments at δ 1.73 ($^2J_{PH}$ = 10.0 Hz), 1.70 ($^2J_{PH}$ = 8.0 Hz), 1.57 ($^2J_{PH}$ = 10.0 Hz) and 1.55 ($^2J_{PH}$ = 8.0 Hz) ppm, each of integral-6. These resonances collapse to the corresponding singlets in the ^{1}H{^{31}P} spectrum. In the ^{1}H NMR spectra there is also a single CH_{cage} resonance of integral two for compound **1** appearing as a doublet δ 2.43 ($^3J_{PH}$ = 14.0 Hz) ppm, confirmed as arising from coupling to phosphorus, since it collapses to a singlet on broad-band ^{31}P decoupling, whilst the CH_{cage} signal of integral two for compound **2** appears at a higher frequency, δ 2.48 ($^3J_{PH}$ = 10.0 Hz) ppm, and collapses to a singlet on broad-band ^{31}P decoupling. Therefore, these two isomers show slightly different characteristics in their proton NMR spectra. Moving to the ^{31}P{^{1}H} NMR spectrum of compound **1**, this shows two mutual doublets with the integral ratio of 1:1 at δ 43.1 and 33.0 ppm and a coupling constant $^2J_{PP}$ = 29.2 Hz. This indicates that in each cage the two phosphorus atoms are magnetically inequivalent. Moreover, the two pairs of phosphorus atoms in different cages are also magnetically equivalent. This clearly shows that the metallacarborane cages are asymmetric. Similarly, the ^{31}P{^{1}H} NMR spectrum of compound **2** reveals two mutually coupled doublets of integral two at δ 43.7

and 33.4 ppm with coupling $^{2}J_{PP}$ = 28.4 Hz, not very different from that of compound **1**. Notably, from the ^{1}H-^{31}P HMBC experiment, the splitting of CH_{cage} arises from the *trans* phosphorus at δ 33.0 ppm for compound **1** and the *trans* phosphorus at δ 33.4 ppm for compound **2**. Therefore, the resonances δ 43.1 ppm and δ 43.7 ppm correspond to the phosphorus atoms *cis* to the CH_{cage} for compound **1** and compound **2**, respectively. The ^{11}B{^{1}H} NMR spectrum of compound **1** consists of seven resonances with relative integrals 2:2:2:2:2:4:4 from high frequency to low frequency, whereas compound **2** shows a distinctly different pattern comprising seven resonances in the integral ratio 2:2:2:2:3:5:2 from high frequency to low frequency. However, this spectroscopic information is not conclusive in determining the exact structures of the *racemic* and *meso* isomers.

A crystallographic study was carried out for both compounds **1** and **2**. It is envisaged that the double deboronation-metalation of 1,1′-bis(*o*-carborane) with {Ni(dmpe)} fragments generates *racemic* and *meso* mixtures with 3,1,2-NiC_2B_9-3′,1′,2′-NiC_2B_9 architectures. Indeed, both cages of compounds **1** and **2** are singly-metalated and in the 3,1,2-NiC_2B_9 form. As regards the identification of the diastereoisomer, a crystallographic C_2 axis passes perpendicular to the C1-C1′ bond, leading to the same chirality for both cages and meaning that compound **1** is a racemic isomer, whereas a non-crystallographic inversion centre *i* can be imagined at the mid-point of the C1-C1′ bond in **2**, meaning different chirality for each cage and showing that compound **2** is a meso isomer. Figure 1 shows a perspective view of a single molecule of *racemic*-[1-(1′-3′-(dmpe)-3′,1′,2′-*closo*-$NiC_2B_9H_{10}$)-3-(dmpe)-3,1,2-*closo*-$NiC_2B_9H_{10}$] (**1**), whereas a perspective view of a single molecule of *meso*-[1-(1′-3′-(dmpe)-3′,1′,2′-*closo*-$NiC_2B_9H_{10}$)-3-(dmpe)-3,1,2-*closo*-$NiC_2B_9H_{10}$] (**2**) is presented in Figure 2. These diastereoisomers are the first such examples in which both the metallacarborane moieties remain unisomerised, i.e.,**1** and **2** are 3,1,2-NiC_2B_9-3′,1′,2′-NiC_2B_9 in racemic and meso forms, previously inaccessible. Both compounds **1** and **2** show clear evidence of internal crowding, since both cages have 3,1,2-NiC_2B_9 architectures. The presence of the {(dmpe)NiC_2B_9} substituents on C1 or C1′ inhibit the free rotation of the {Ni(dmpe)} fragment on both the primed and non-primed cages. It is confirmed that in each cage the phosphorus atoms are inequivalent, giving rise to two doublets observed in the ^{31}P NMR spectra (previously discussed). Since both cages are of the 3,1,2-NiC_2B_9 form, the two metallacarborane units at C1 and C1′ push each other away, so that the {Ni(dmpe)} fragment is bent away from its ideal orientation within the cages. In principle, the ideal orientation of the {NiP1P2} fragment in a NiC_2B_9 icosahedron is perpendicular to the vertical mirror plane through the C_2B_9 unit, conveniently defined by the interplane dihedral angle (θ) of 90°. [8] For compound **1**, θ is found to be 55.36(8)° for both the primed cage and non-primed cage, whilst for compound **2**, θ is 57.59(15)° and 49.58(18)° for the primed cage and the non-primed cage, respectively. These were calculated using the planes through Ni3P1P2 and Ni3′P1′P2′ and through B6B8B10 and B6′B8′B10′for the non-primed and primed cages, respectively. Thus, the dihedral angles are clearly twisted away from the idealised 90°. We also note that in compound **1** the {NiPP} plane is bent away from the perpendicular to the bottom pentagonal B5B6B11B12B9 plane by.6(7)°, whereas in compound **2** the corresponding angles are 6.1(12)° for the non-primed cage and 21.5(15)° for the primed cage. The internal steric crowding between two (dmpe)NiC_2B_9 units is also evidenced by the elongated Ni3-C1 distances compared to Ni3–C2 [compound **1** primed cage: 2.2977(19) *versus* 2.0657(18) Å]. This is also evidenced in compound **2**, Ni3-C1: 2.326(4) [Ni2-C2: 2.066(4) Å] and Ni3′-C1′: 2.299(4) [Ni2′-C2′: 2.103(3) Å].

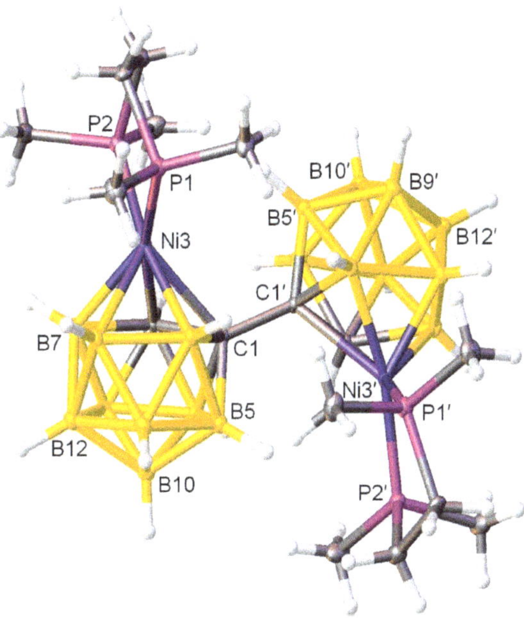

Figure 1. Molecular structure of *rac*-[1-(1′-3′-(dmpe)-3′,1′,2′-*closo*-$NiC_2B_9H_{10}$)-3-(dmpe)-3,1,2-*closo*-$NiC_2B_9H_{10}$] (**1**). Atoms with dashed suffixes are generated by the symmetry operation 1.5-x, y, 0.5-z.

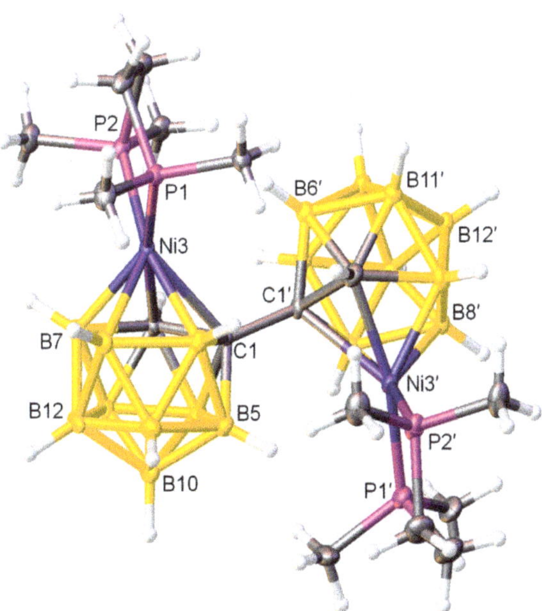

Figure 2. Molecular structure of *meso*-[1-(1′-3′-(dmpe)-3′,1′,2′-*closo*-$NiC_2B_9H_{10}$)-3-(dmpe)-3,1,2-*closo*-$NiC_2B_9H_{10}$] (**2**).

3.2. Characterisation of Compounds 3 and 4α

The treatment of $[Tl]_2[1\text{-}(1'\text{-}3',1',2'\text{-}closo\text{-}TlC_2B_9H_{10})\text{-}3,1,2\text{-}closo\text{-}TlC_2B_9H_{10}]$ in THF with $[Ni(dppe)Cl_2]$ at room temperature followed by work up and purification involving preparative TLC afforded two army-green bands, compounds **3** and **4α** (Scheme 3). The compounds were characterised spectroscopically as well as by single crystal XRD.

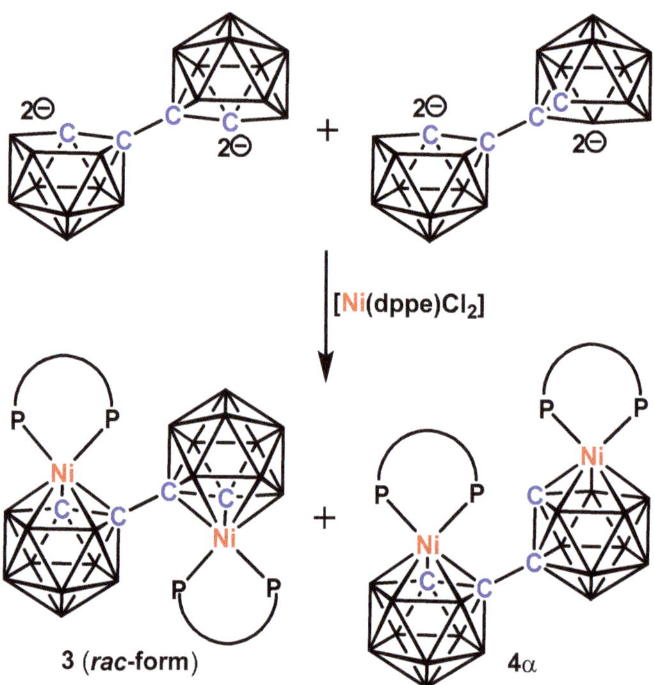

Scheme 3. Synthesis of **3** and **4α** from the nickelation of $[Tl]_2[1\text{-}(1'\text{-}3',1',2'\text{-}closo\text{-}TlC_2B_9H_{10})\text{-}3,1,2\text{-}closo\text{-}TlC_2B_9H_{10}]$. NiPP = {Ni(dppe)}.

Earlier we noted a diastereoisomeric mixture resulting from the deboronation-metalation of 1,1′-bis(*o*-carborane) with the {Ni(dmpe)} fragment. However, with the {Ni(dppe)} fragment, additionally, isomerisation occurred in the case of a mono-metalated $[3,1,2\text{-}(dppe)\text{-}NiC_2B_9\text{-}1,2\text{-}C_2B_{10}]$ species which transformed to $[4,1,2\text{-}(dppe)\text{-}NiC_2B_9\text{-}1,2\text{-}C_2B_{10}]$ due to the stereo-electronic nature of the dppe. [8] Therefore, with double metalation using the{Ni(dppe)} fragment, the products could be diastereoisomers, stereospecific products and other isomers thereof. Although the ^1H NMR spectra of **3** and **4α** are more complex than those of compounds **1** and **2**, there are resonances from phenyl protons and methylene bridge protons of the dppe. In the proton spectrum of **3**, there is also a CH_{cage} resonance of integral two which appears at δ 1.84 ppm as a doublet J = 11.6 Hz, whilst in the proton spectrum of **4α**, there are two CH_{cage} resonances, each of integral-1, one at δ 1.94 ppm appearing as a singlet and the other at δ 1.67 ppm appearing as a doublet J = 11.2 Hz. The doublets collapse to singlets in the $^1H\{^{31}P\}$ spectra. Notably the CH_{cage} resonance of **3** appears at a lower frequency than that of **1** (δ 2.43 ppm) or **2** (δ 2.48 ppm). The two doublet CH_{cage} resonances clearly indicate that both cages of compound **3** are nickellated and could be of $3,1,2\text{-}NiC_2B_9\text{-}3',1',2'\text{-}NiC_2B_9$ architecture with reference to the proton spectra of compounds **1** and **2**. The doublet and singlet CH_{cage} resonances indicate that nickelation occurred for both cages of compound **4α** where one cage could be unisomerised, i.e., the $\{3,1,2\text{-}NiC_2B_9\}$ form and another cage could be isomerised to either a $\{4,1,2\text{-}NiC_2B_9\}$ or a $\{2,1,8\text{-}NiC_2B_9\}$ form. These inferences are further supported by the ^{31}P NMR spectra of compounds **3** and **4α**. The $^{31}P\{^1H\}$ NMR spectrum of compound **3** consists of two mutual doublets with integral ratio 1:1 at δ 51.6 and 39.2 ppm with coupling J = 19.1 Hz; on the contrary, the $^{31}P\{^1H\}$ NMR spectrum of **4α** consists of a singlet of integral-2 at δ 62.9 ppm and two mutual doublets, each of integral-1 at δ 49.4 and 47.5 ppm, with a coupling J = 16.6 Hz. This signifies the asymmetric nature of each metallacarborane cage but the symmetric nature of the whole molecule. The $^{11}B\{^1H\}$ spectrum of compound **3** reveals five resonances with the relative integrals 2:4:2:5:5 from high frequency to low frequency, a different pattern to that for compounds **1** or **2**, whilst the $^{11}B\{^1H\}$ NMR spectrum of **4α** consists of multiple overlapping resonances with a total integral of 18B and is different in pattern to that of compounds **1**, **2** and **3**, thus preventing the identification of the exact isomer present and thereby requiring single crystal XRD analysis.

The precise natures of **3** and **4α** were confirmed by crystallographic analysis. The racemic form of compound **3** is confirmed by a crystallographic C_2 axis passing through the mid-point of the C1-C1′ bond, and thus requiring both cages to be of the same chirality. Figure 3 shows a perspective view of a single molecule of *rac*-[1-(1′-3′-(dppe)-3′,1′,2′-*closo*-$NiC_2B_9H_{10}$)-3-(dppe)-3,1,2-*closo*-$NiC_2B_9H_{10}$] (**3**). However, it is clear that for compound **4α** one of the cages has isomerised. A perspective view of a single molecule of [1-(2′-4′-(dppe)-4′,1′,2′-*closo*-$NiC_2B_9H_{10}$)-3-(dppe)-3,1,2-*closo*-$NiC_2B_9H_{10}$] (**4α**) is shown in Figure 4. For compound **3**, both cages are nickellated by {Ni(dppe)} fragments and are of 3,1,2-NiC_2B_9 architecture. As noted, the midpoint of the C1-C1′ bond lies on a crystallographic 2-fold axis. This leads to two bulky {(dppe)NiC_2B_9} units, connected at C1 and C1′, pushing each other apart. There is a clear indication of internal crowding which is obvious from the orientation of the {NiP1P2} fragment in the NiC_2B_9 icosahedra. In **3** (for the non-primed cage), the θ (previously discussed) between the plane containing Ni3P1P2 and the plane through B6B8B10 is 60.72(9)°, which deviates significantly from 90°. Further evidence of steric congestion is demonstrated by the fact that the plane of the {NiP1P2} fragment deviates from perpendicularity to the plane through B5B6B11B12B9 vertices by 6.6(8)°. Additionally, the longer Ni3–C1 distance compared to Ni3–C2 [2.336(2) *versus* 2.124(2) Å] again supports significant steric crowding in the molecule. The steric congestion in **3** would be slightly relieved if the 3,1,2-NiC_2B_9 cage would isomerise to either the 4,1,2-NiC_2B_9 form or the 2,1,8-NiC_2B_9 form. Indeed, this has been experimentally observed in **4α**, which is of 3,1,2-NiC_2B_9-4′,1′,2′-NiC_2B_9 form, where one of the cages has isomerised. The molecule of **4α** is partly disordered (two orientations for a phenyl ring), but the atomic connectivity is nonetheless clear. The internal crowding slightly reduces as, for compound **4α** (for 3,1,2-NiC_2B_9 cage), the θ between the Ni3P1P2 and B6B8B10 planes is 64.8(4)°, closer to the idealised 90°. However, in **4α**, the non-primed (3,1,2-NiC_2B_9 cage) still has significant internal crowding, as indicated by the longer distances Ni3-C1: 2.327(9) Å *versus* Ni2-C2: 2.129(9) Å. The relaxation of steric congestion in the (4′,1′,2′-NiC_2B_9 cage) of **4α** is reflected in the slightly shorter distance Ni4′-C1′ is 2.167(8) Å. Furthermore the dihedral angle between the Ni4′P1′P2′ and C1′B11′B12′ planes for the primed cage is 86.1(4)°. Thus, the metalation of doubly deboronated species from 1,1′-bis(*o*-carborane) with {Ni(dppe)} results in bis-nickelated products, and although in principle both *racemic* and *meso* products were anticipated, only stereospecific racemic-**3** and **4α** were observed. The meso form was not found. The rationale for the formation of the *rac* form is discussed below.

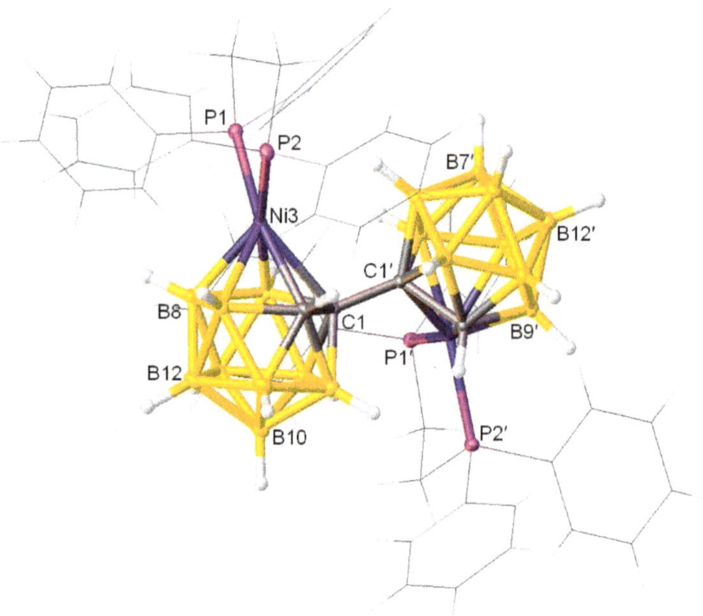

Figure 3. A perspective view of *rac*-[1-(1′-3′-(dppe)-3′,1′,2′-*closo*-$NiC_2B_9H_{10}$)-3-(dppe)-3,1,2-*closo*-$NiC_2B_9H_{10}$] (**3**) (all phenyls and the $–CH_2–CH_2–$ bridge of dppe are in wireframe for clarity). Atoms with dashed suffixes are generated by the symmetry operation 1 − x, y, 0.5 − z.

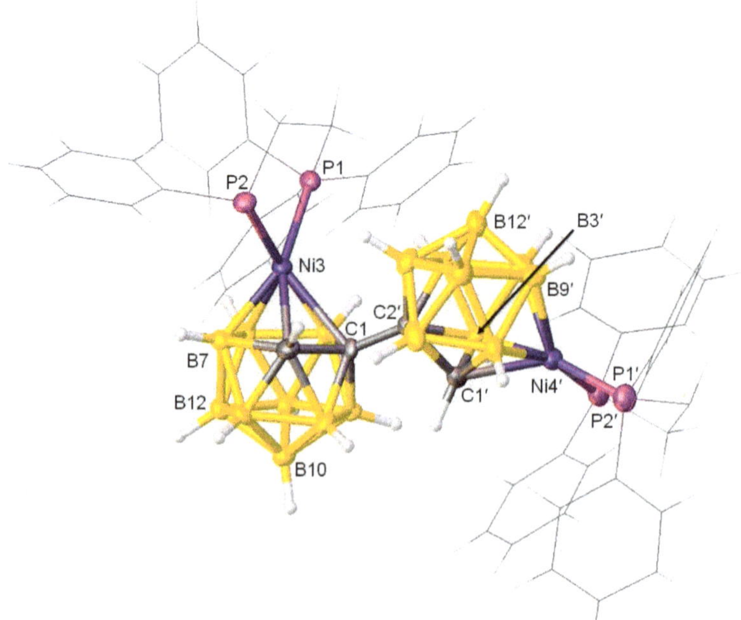

Figure 4. Molecular structure of [1-(2′-4′-(dppe)-4′,1′,2′-*closo*-$NiC_2B_9H_{10}$)-3-(dppe)-3,1,2-*closo*-$NiC_2B_9H_{10}$] (**4α**) (all phenyls and the $–CH_2$-CH_2- bridge of dppe are in wireframe for clarity).

3.3. Dihydrogen Interaction in 3 and Isomerisation in 4α

The reaction of the [7-(7′-7′,8′-*nido*-$C_2B_9H_{10}$)-7,8-*nido*-$C_2B_9H_{10}]^{4-}$ tetraanion with {Ni(dmpe)} fragments affords diastereomeric mixture products, i.e., *rac* (**1**) and *meso* (**2**) forms of 3,1,2-NiC_2B_9-3′,1′,2′-NiC_2B_9, whereas the same reaction with the more bulky {Ni(dppe)} fragment results in two isolable stereospecific products, i.e., *rac* 3,1,2-NiC_2B_9-3′,1′,2′-NiC_2B_9 (**3**) and 3,1,2-NiC_2B_9-4′,1′,2′-NiC_2B_9, in compound **4α**. The isolated *rac*-**3** displays intramolecular dihydrogen bonding, as was found previously during the rationalisation of the stereospecific {CoCp} fragment metalation reaction with the [7-(7′-7′,8′-*nido*-$C_2B_9H_{10}$)-7,8-*nido*-$C_2B_9H_{10}]^{4-}$ tetranion to form the only racemic form of the product 3,1,2-CoC_2B_9-3′,1′,2′-CoC_2B_9 [9]. The formation of intramolecular dihydrogen bonding associated with C*H* atoms of one cage and B*H* atoms of the other cage results from the relatively protonic and hydridic nature of the C*H* and B*H* atoms, respectively. ^{11}B NMR analysis of individual vertices for 3,1,2-MC_2B_9 compounds established that the most hydridic B*H* atoms are H5 and H6 [18]. In the case of *rac*-**3**, the orientation of two {(dppe)NiC_2B_9} cages enables two sets of intramolecular dihydrogen bonds, CH2$\cdots$BH6^{i} 2.07(3) Å (where i = 1 − x, y, 0.5 − z) and its symmetry equivalent, CH2$^{i}\cdots$BH6. Notably, the hypothetical analogous meso form could only allow for one set of such intramolecular dihydrogen bonding, whatever the rotameric arrangement, thereby rendering the *meso* isomer less favourable.

Crowding between the bulky {(dppe)(3,1,2-NiC_2B_9)} substituent on C1′ and the dppe ligand on Ni3 of an unisomerised 3,1,2-NiC_2B_9-3′,1′,2′-NiC_2B_9 species is likely to be the major cause of the isomerisation observed in compound **4α**. Isomerisation moves the {(dppe)(3,1,2-NiC_2B_9)} substituent down to the lower pentagonal belt further away from the {Ni(dppe)$_2$} on the other cage. Indeed, we have already observed steric crowding in the unisomerised compound **3**. In regards to the {3′,1′,2′-NiC_2B_9} to {4′,1′,2′-NiC_2B_9} isomerisation, this can likely be related to electronic factors, specifically the electron withdrawing nature of the dppe ligand. A similar 3,1,2- to 4,1,2- isomerisation of mono-metalated nickelacarboranes with dppe and PPh_2Me ligands has been previously established [8].

4. Conclusions

Four new bis(nickelated) species are documented from the metalation of doubly deboronated 1,1′-bis(*o*-carborane), and their identity was confirmed by both spectroscopic and crystallographic means. The metalation of the {Ni(dmpe)} fragment with the Tl_4-salt gives diastereoisomeric products with the unusual crowded architecture of 3,1,2-NiC_2B_9-3′,1′,2′-NiC_2B_9 as racemic and meso forms. In contrast, metalation with the {Ni(dppe)} fragment results in the 3,1,2-NiC_2B_9-4′,1′,2′-NiC_2B_9 species, a stereospecific racemic product. The racemic product in the latter case shows intramolecular dihydrogen bonding, hence explaining the stereospecific reaction, whereas the stereo-electronic nature of the bis(phosphine) ligand influences the formation of the isomerised 3,1,2-NiC_2B_9-4′,1′,2′-NiC_2B_9 species.

Supplementary Materials: The following are available online at https://www.mdpi.com/2073-4352/11/1/16/s1, NMR spectra of all new compounds are available online along with the crystallographic data, free of charge. Crystallographic information for all compounds here has been deposited in the Cambridge Crystallographic Data Centre as supplementary publications nos. CCDC 2048463, 2048465, 2,048,466 and 2,048,464 (compounds **1**, **2**, **3** and **4α**).

Author Contributions: Syntheses and original draft preparation, and editing, D.M.; final structure analysis and manuscript editing, G.M.R. All authors have read and agreed to the published version of the manuscript.

Funding: D.M. is grateful to the Heriot-Watt University for financial assistance; a James-Watt Ph.D. studentship was awarded to D.M. from 2013 to 2016. We thank EPSRC for funding the Bruker X8Apex2 diffractometer.

Institutional Review Board Statement: Not applicable.

Informed Consent Statement: Not applicable.

Data Availability Statement: Not applicable.

Acknowledgments: This work is taken from the Ph.D. thesis (2016) of D.M., supervised by Alan J. Welch at Heriot-Watt University. We thank EPSRC for funding the Bruker X8Apex2 diffractometer and the U.K. National Crystallography Service for data collection of compound **4**α.

Conflicts of Interest: The authors declare no conflict of interest.

References

1. Sivaev, I.B.; Bregadze, V.I. 1,1′-Bis(*ortho*-carborane)-based transition metal complexes. *Co-ord. Chem. Rev.* **2019**, *392*, 146–176. [CrossRef]
2. Yruegas, S.; Axtell, J.C.; Kirlikovali, K.O.; Spokoyny, A.M.; Martin, C.D. Synthesis of 9-borafluorene analogues featuring a three-dimensional 1,1′-bis (*o*-carborane) backbone. *Chem. Commun.* **2019**, *55*, 2892–2895. [CrossRef] [PubMed]
3. Jeans, R.J.; Chan, A.P.Y.; Riley, L.E.; Taylor, J.; Rosair, G.M.; Welch, A.J.; Sivaev, I.B. Arene-Ruthenium complexes of 1,1′-bis (ortho-carborane): Synthesis, characterization, and catalysis. *Inorg. Chem.* **2019**, *58*, 11751–11761. [CrossRef] [PubMed]
4. Chan, A.P.Y.; Parkinson, J.A.; Rosair, G.M.; Welch, A.J. Bis (phosphine) hydridorhodacarborane derivatives of 1,1′-bis (*ortho*-carborane) and their catalysis of alkene isomerization and the hydrosilylation of acetophenone. *Inorg. Chem.* **2020**, *59*, 2011–2023. [CrossRef] [PubMed]
5. Kirlikovali, K.O.; Axtell, J.C.; Anderson, K.P.; Djurovich, P.I.; Rheingold, A.L.; Spokoyny, A.M. Fine-tuning electronic properties of luminescent Pt (II) complexes via vertex-differentiated coordination of sterically invariant carborane-based ligands. *Organometallics* **2018**, *37*, 3122–3131. [CrossRef]
6. Wu, J.; Cao, K.; Zhang, C.-Y.; Xu, T.-T.; Ding, L.-F.; Li, B.; Yang, J. Catalytic oxidative dehydrogenative coupling of cage B–H/B–H bonds for synthesis of bis (o-carborane)s. *Org. Lett.* **2019**, *21*, 5986–5989. [CrossRef] [PubMed]
7. Thiripuranathar, G.; Man, W.Y.; Palmero, C.; Chan, A.P.Y.; Leube, B.T.; Ellis, D.; McKay, D.; MacGregor, S.A.; Jourdan, L.; Rosair, G.M.; et al. Icosahedral metallacarborane/carborane species derived from 1,1′-bis(*o*-carborane). *Dalton Trans.* **2015**, *44*, 5628–5637. [CrossRef] [PubMed]
8. Mandal, D.; Man, W.Y.; Rosair, G.M.; Welch, A.J. Steric versus electronic factors in metallacarborane isomerisation: Nickelacarboranes with 3,1,2-, 4,1,2- and 2,1,8-NiC 2 B 9 architectures and pendant carborane groups, derived from 1,1′-bis(o-carborane). *Dalton Trans.* **2016**, *45*, 15013–15025. [CrossRef] [PubMed]
9. Thiripuranathar, G.; Mandal, D.; Argentari, M.; Chan, A.P.Y.; Man, W.Y.; Rosair, G.M.; Welch, A.J. Double deboronation and homometalation of 1,1′-bis (*ortho*-carborane). *Dalton Trans.* **2017**, *46*, 1811–1821. [CrossRef] [PubMed]
10. Behnken, P.E.; Marder, T.B.; Baker, R.T.; Knobler, C.B.; Thompson, M.R.; Hawthorne, M.F. Synthesis, structural characterization, and stereospecificity in the formation of bimetallic rhodacarborane clusters containing rhodium-hydrogen-boron bridge interactions. *J. Am. Chem. Soc.* **1985**, *107*, 932–940. [CrossRef]
11. Chan, A.P.Y.; Rosair, G.M.; Welch, A.J. Heterometalation of 1,1′-bis (ortho-carborane). *Inorg. Chem.* **2018**, *57*, 8002–8011. [CrossRef] [PubMed]
12. Ren, S.; Xie, Z. A facile and practical synthetic route to 1,1′-bis (*o*-carborane). *Organometallics* **2008**, *27*, 5167–5168. [CrossRef]
13. Booth, G.; Chatt, J. 590. Some complexes of ditertiary phosphines with nickel (II) and nickel (III). *J. Chem. Soc.* **2004**, 3238–3241. [CrossRef]
14. Bruker AXS. *APEX2-Software Suite for Crystallographic Programs;* Bruker AXS, Inc.: Madison, WI, USA, 2009.
15. Sheldrick, G.M. A short history of SHELX. *Acta. Cryst.* **2008**, *A64*, 112–122. [CrossRef] [PubMed]
16. Dolomanov, O.V.; Bourhis, L.J.; Gildea, R.J.; Howard, J.A.K.; Puschmann, H. OLEX2: A complete structure solution, refinement and analysis program. *J. Appl. Crystallogr.* **2009**, *42*, 339–341. [CrossRef]
17. McAnaw, A.; Scott, G.; Elrick, L.; Rosair, G.M.; Welch, A.J. The VCD method-A simple and reliable way to distinguish cage C and B atoms in (hetero) carborane structures determined crystallographically. *Dalton Trans.* **2013**, *42*, 645–664. [CrossRef] [PubMed]
18. Bown, M.; Plešek, J.; Baše, K.; Štibr, B.; Fontaine, X.L.R.; Greenwood, N.N.; Kennedy, J.D. Assigned cluster ^{11}B and ^{1}H NMR properties of [3-(η6-C6Me6)-closo-3,1,2-RuC2B9H11]. *Magn. Reson. Chem.* **1989**, *27*, 947–949. [CrossRef]

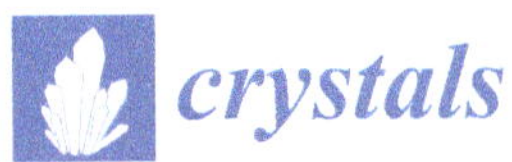

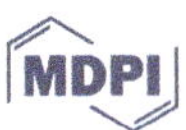

Article

"Free of Base" Sulfa-Michael Addition for Novel *o*-Carboranyl-DL-Cysteine Synthesis †

Julia Laskova [1,*], Irina Kosenko [1], Ivan Ananyev [1], Marina Stogniy [1,2], Igor Sivaev [1] and Vladimir Bregadze [1]

1 A.N.Nesmeyanov Institute of Organoelement Compounds, Russian Academy of Sciences, Vavilova str. 28, 119991 Moscow, Russia; ira.kosenko@gmail.com (I.K.); i.ananyev@gmail.com (I.A.); stogniymarina@rambler.ru (M.S.); sivaev@ineos.ac.ru (I.S.); bre@ineos.ac.ru (V.B.)

2 M.V. Lomonosov Institute of Fine Chemical Technology, MIREA—Russian Technological University, 86 Vernadsky Av., 119571 Moscow, Russia

* Correspondence: laskova@ineos.ac.ru; Tel.: +7-905-551-8846

† Dedicated to Professor Alan J. Welch in recognition of his outstanding contribution in the chemistry of carboranes.

Received: 2 November 2020; Accepted: 7 December 2020; Published: 11 December 2020

Abstract: The sulfa-Michael addition reaction was applied for the two-step synthesis of *o*-carboranyl cysteine 1-$HOOCCH(NH_2)CH_2S$-1,2-$C_2B_{10}H_{11}$ from the trimethylammonium salt of 1-mercapto-*o*-carborane and methyl 2-acetamidoacrylate. To avoid the decapitation of o-carborane into its *nido*-form, the "free of base" method under mild conditions in a system of two immiscible solvents toluene-H_2O was developed. The replacement of H_2O by ^2H_2O resulted in carboranyl-cysteine containing a deuterium label at the α-position of the amino acid 1-$HOOCCD(NH_2)CH_2S$-1,2-$C_2B_{10}H_{11}$. The structure of the protected *o*-carboranyl cysteine was determined by single-crystal X-ray diffraction. The obtained compounds can be considered as potential agents for the Boron Neutron Capture Therapy of cancer.

Keywords: boron chemistry; *o*-carborane; sulfa-Michael addition reaction; cysteine; boron neutron capture therapy; *o*-carborane decapitation; labeled compound

---

1. Introduction

Cancer remains one of the major health issues and the second leading cause of death worldwide [1]. Radiation therapy has a central role in the management of malignant brain tumors, especially for the most aggressive ones [2–4]. First introduced in 1936 by Locher [5], the Boron Neutron Capture Therapy model (BNCT) is a promising type of radiation therapy for cancer that has the potential to be an important treatment for numerous types of tumors, including for those lying in areas that are difficult to access for surgery intervention, such as high-grade gliomas and metastatic brain tumors [6–8] Currently, only two low molecular weight boron-containing compounds, sodium mercapto-undecahydro-*closo*-dodecaborate (BSH, developed in about 1965) and a water-soluble fructose complex of borylphenylalanine (BPA, discovered in 1958), have been approved and found clinical use in BNCT [9–11].

Recent advances in the development of potential agents for BNCT treatment include various boron-containing bioconjugates [12]; there are many with natural and unnatural amino acids among them [13]. It is believed that amino acid conjugates are preferentially taken up by rapidly growing tumor cells [14]. Polyhedral carboranes as a boron-rich compounds are considered to have potential for usage in BNCT [15]. In this regard, the chemistry of dicarbaboranes [$C_2B_{10}H_{12}$] and their derivatives has been well investigated [16]. The synthesis of *o*-carboranes containing unnatural ω-mercapto-amino acids with side-chain lengths ranging from 4 to 6 methylene units **1(a–c)** [17], L-*o*-carboranyl-alanine

2 [18] as well as *o*-carboranyl derivatives of (S)-Asparagine **3a** and (S)-Glutamine **3b** [19], phenylalanine **4** [20] and (S)-*m*-carboranyl-homocysteine sulfoxide **5** [21], have been published. Our current interest was inspired by the recent synthesis [22] of *m*-carboranyl-cysteine **6** and its biological evaluation as an agent for Boron Neutron Capture Therapy [23,24] (Figure 1). Therefore, we decided to synthesize its analogue based on readily available 1-mercapto-*o*-carborane [25,26].

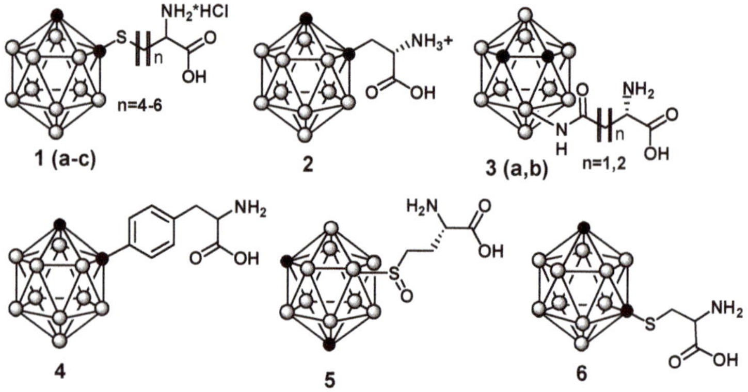

Figure 1. *o*- and *m*- carborane–amino acid conjugates.

Here, we report the synthesis of *o*-carboranyl-cysteine via the sulfa-Michael addition reaction of an easily available salt of 1-mercapto-*o*-carborane and methyl 2-acetamidoacrylate (MAA) using a two-phase system.

2. Materials and Methods

2.1. General

$[1\text{-S-}1,2\text{-}C_2B_{10}H_{11}](Me_3NH)$ (**7**) was prepared according to the literature procedure [27]. Methyl 2-acetamidoacrylate (Sigma Aldrich Chemie GmbH, NJ, USA) was used without purification. ^2H_2O was received from Carl Roth GmbH. The reaction proceedings were monitored via thin-layer chromatograms (Merck F254 silica gel on aluminums plates). Boron compounds were visualized with $PdCl_2$ stain solution, which, upon heating, gave dark brown spots. Purifications were carried out using column chromatography with Silica gel 60 0.060–0.200 mm (Acros Organics, NJ, USA). ^1H, ^{13}C, and ^{11}B NMR spectra were recorded at 400.13, 100.61, and 128.38 MHz, respectively, on a BRUKER-Avance-400 spectrometer. Tetramethylsilane and $BF_3 \times Et_2O$ were used as standards for ^1H, ^{13}C NMR, and ^{11}B NMR, respectively. All the chemical shifts are reported in ppm (δ) relative to external standards. IR spectra were recorded on an IR Prestige-21 (SHIMADZU, Kyoto, Japan) instrument. High-resolution mass spectra (HRMS) were measured on a Bruker micrOTOF II instrument using electrospray ionization (ESI), with a mass range from *m*/*z* 50 to *m*/*z* 3000; external or internal calibration was carried out with ESI Tuning Mix, Agilent. Spectra can be found in the Supplementary Materials.

2.2. Synthesis of $1\text{-}CH_3O(O)C(CH_3(O)CHN)CHCH_2S\text{-}1,2\text{-}C_2B_{10}H_{11}$ (8)

To a solution of **7** (0.5 g, 2.1 mmol) in toluene (30 mL) methyl 2-acetamidoacrylate (0.3 g, 2.1 mmol) and H_2O (30 mL) were added; the resulting system was vigorously stirred under reflux for 24 h. Then, the mixture was cooled to r.t. and the toluene layer was separated, washed with H_2O (2 × 20), dried over Na_2SO_4, and evaporated. The product was purified by silica gel column chromatography using Et_2O as an eluent and vacuum-dried to give a light yellow solid. Yield: 0.46 g (68%). ^1H NMR (Chloroform-*d*) δ = 6.29 (d, *J* = 7.7 Hz, 1H, NH), 4.89 (td, *J* = 7.2, 4.5 Hz, 1H, α-CH), 3.99 (broad s, 1H, carb-CH), 3.82 (s, 3H, $COOCH_3$), 3.51 (dd, *J* = 13.4, 4.6 Hz, 1H, CH_2CH), 3.18 (dd, *J* = 13.4,

6.9 Hz, 1H, CH_2CH), 2.06 (s, 3H, NHCOCH_3), 3.0–1.5 (broad, 10H, BH); ^{11}B NMR (Chloroform-*d*) δ = −1.5 (d, *J* = 150 Hz, 1B), −4.7 (d, *J* = 146 Hz, 1B), −8.8 (d, *J* = 154 Hz, 4B), −12.2 (d, *J* = 162 Hz, 4B); ^{13}C NMR (Chloroform-*d*) δ = 170.21, 170.17 (CO), 73.9, 67.9 (C-carb), 53.2 (OCH_3), 51.2 (α-CH), 39.4 (CH_2CH), 23.1 ($COCH_3$). ESI-MS, *m/z*, $C_8H_{21}B_{10}NO_3S$ calcd. 320.2322, found 320.2322 ([M+H]$^+$). IR-FT (ν, cm^{-1}): 3371(NH), 3060 (CH-carb); 2948, 2926, 2852 (broad CH); 2607, 2584, 2557 (BH); 1736, 16177 (CO).

2.3. Synthesis of 1-HOOC(NH_2)CHCH_2S-1,2-$C_2B_{10}H_{11}$ × HCl (9)

Water (2 mL) and concentrated HCl (10 mL) were added to a solution of **8** (0.1 g, 0.3 mmol) in glacial acetic acid (10 mL). The resulting mixture was heated at 70 °C for 40 h., cooled to r.t., and evaporated. The residue was suspended in 5 mL of water, formed solid was filtered, washed with water (2 × 5 mL) and vacuum dried to give **9**. Light yellow solid (0.093 mg, 70%). ^{1}H NMR (Methanol-*d4*) δ = 4.89 (s, 1H, carb-CH), 4.09 (m, 1H, α-CH), 3.64 (m, 1H, CH_2CH), 3.43 (m, 1H, CH_2CH), 3.0–1.5 (broad, 10H, BH); ^{11}B NMR (Methanol-d_4) δ = −1.8 (d, *J* = 151 Hz, 1B), −5.1 (d, *J* = 148 Hz, 1B), −9.2 (d, *J* = 148 Hz, 4B), −12.3 (d, *J* = 172 Hz, 4B). ^{13}C NMR (Methanol-d_4) δ 172.0 (COOH), 74.8, 68.4 (C-carb), 51.60 (α-CH), 38.3 (CH_2CH). ESI-MS, *m/z*, C5H17B10NO2S calcd. 264.2059, found 264.2061. IR-FT (ν, cm^{-1}): 3399 (broad NH$^+$), 3058 (CH- carb); 2923, 2854 (CH); 2580 (broad BH), 1728 (CO).

2.4. Synthesis of 1-CH_3O(O)C(CH_3(O)CHN)CDCH_2S-1,2-$C_2B_{10}H_{11}$ (10)

Under an argon atmosphere, methyl 2-acetamidoacrylate (0.06 g, 0.4 mmol) and ^2H_2O (5 mL) were added to a solution of **7** (0.1 g, 0.4 mmol) in toluene (15 mL); the resulting two-phase system was vigorously stirred under reflux for 30 h. Purification was held in the same manner as for compound **8**. Light yellow solid (90 mg, 66%). ^{1}H NMR (Chloroform-*d*) δ = 6.31 (s, 1H, NH), 4.00 (broad s, 1H, CH-carb), 3.82 (s, 3H, $COOCH_3$), 3.50 (d, *J* = 13.4 Hz, 1H, CH_2CD), 3.17 (d, *J* = 13.4 Hz, 1H, CH_2CD), 2.06 (s, 3H, NHCOCH_3), 3.0–1.5 (broad, 10H, BH); ^{11}B NMR (Chloroform-*d*) δ = −1.5 (d, *J* = 151 Hz, 1B), −4.8 (d, *J* = 150 Hz, 1B), −8.9 (d, *J* = 151 Hz, 4B), −12.4 (d, *J* = 176 Hz, 4B); ^{13}C NMR (Chloroform-*d*) δ = 170.23, 170.17 (CO), 73.9, 67.9 (C-carb), 53.2 (OCH_3), 51.0 (t, α-CD), 39.3 (CH_2), 23.1 ($COCH_3$). ESI-MS, *m/z*, $C_8H_{20}DB_{10}NO_3S$ calcd. 321.2385, found 321.2399. IR-FT (ν, cm^{-1}): 3370 (NH), 3061 (CH- carb); 2953 (CH); 2608, 2586, 2557 (BH), 1733, 1674 (CO).

2.5. Synthesis of 1-HOOC(NH_2)CDCH_2S-1,2-$C_2B_{10}H_{11}$ × HCl (11)

Water (2 mL) and concentrated HCl (5 mL) were added to a solution of **10** (0.05 g, 0.16 mmol) in glacial acetic acid (5 mL). The resulting mixture was heated at 70 °C for 40 h., cooled to r.t., and evaporated. The residue was suspended in 5 mL of water, formed solid was filtered, washed with water (2 mL) and vacuum dried to yield **11**: 38 mg (81%). ^{1}H NMR (Methanol-d_4) δ = 4.88 (broad s, 1H, CH-carb), 4.27–4.20 (α-CH, m, 0,1H), 3.64 (d, *J* = 13.9 Hz, 1H, CH_2CD), 3.44 (d, *J* = 13.9 Hz, 1H, CH_2CD), 3.0–1.5 (broad, 10H, BH). ^{11}B NMR (Methanol-d_4) δ = -1.9 (d, *J* = 149 Hz, 1B), −4.9 (d, *J* = 140 Hz, 1B), −9.0 (d, *J* = 143 Hz, 4B), −12.3 (d, *J* = 175 Hz, 4B). ^{13}C NMR (Methanol-d_4) δ = 168.0 (CO), 73.6 (C-carb), 68.4 (C-carb), 51.8 (α-C), 36.0 (CH_2). ESI-MS, *m/z*, $C_5H_{17}B_{10}NO_2S$ calcd. 265.2122, found 265.2127.

2.6. Synthesis of 1-CH_3O(O)C(CH_3(O)CHN)CHCH_2S-2-D-1,2-$C_2B_{10}H_{10}$ (12)

Under an argon atmosphere, methyl 2-acetamidoacrylate (0.06 g, 0.4 mmol), ^2H_2O (5 mL), and anhydrous K_2CO_3 (0.055 g, 0.4 mmol) were added to a solution of **7** (0.1 g, 0.4 mmol) in toluene (15 mL); the resulting system was vigorously stirred under reflux for 10 h. The purification was held in the same manner as for compound **8**. Light yellow solid (13 mg, 10%). ^{1}H NMR (Chloroform-*d*) δ = 6.20 (d, *J* = 7.7 Hz, 1H, NH), 4.90 (td, *J* = 7.2, 4.7 Hz, 1H, α-CH), 4.00 (undetectable, s, 0H, carb-CD), 3.83 (s, 3H, $COOCH_3$), 3.53 (dd, *J* = 13.4, 4.7 Hz, 1H, CH_2CH), 3.19 (dd, *J* = 13.4, 6.9 Hz, 1H, CH_2CH), 2.07 (s, 3H, NHCOCH_3), 3.0–1.5 (broad, 10H, BH); ^{11}B NMR (Chloroform-*d*) δ = −1.5 (d, *J* = 152 Hz, 1B), −4.8 (d, *J* = 147 Hz, 1B), −8.9 (d, *J* = 152 Hz, 4B), −12.5 (d, *J* = 173 Hz, 4B); ^{13}C NMR (Chloroform-*d*) δ = 170.16,170.14 (CO), 73.8 (CH-carb), 68.5–66.8 (t, CD-carb), 53.2 (OCH_3), 51.2

(α-CH), 39.4 (CH_2), 23.1 ($COCH_3$). ESI-MS, *m/z*, $C_8H_{20}DB_{10}NO_3S$ calcd. 321.2385, found 321.2384. IR-FT (ν, cm^{-1}): 3372(NH), 2923, 2851 (CH); 2607, 2584, 2557 (BH); 2289 (CD-carb); 1736, 1677 (CO).

2.7. X-ray Diffraction

Crystals of **8** are triclinic, space group P-1, at 120K: a = 7.6513(5), b = 10.5669(7), c = 11.5392(7), α= 68.378(1)°, β = 85.686(1)°, γ = 72.663(1)°, V = 827.27(9) $Å^3$, Z = 2 (Z′ = 1), d_{calc} = 1.282 g·cm^{-3}, F(000) = 332. Intensities of 11,058 reflections were measured with a Bruker SMART APEX 2 Duo CCD diffractometer [λ(MoKα) = 0.71072Å, ω-scans, 2θ < 60°] and 4824 independent reflections [R_{int} = 0.0324] were used in further refinement. The structure was solved by the direct method and refined by the full-matrix least-squares technique against F^2 in the anisotropic-isotropic approximation. The hydrogen atoms were found in the difference Fourier synthesis and refined in the isotropic approximation within the riding model. For **8**, the refinement converged to wR_2 = 0.1167 and GOF = 0.781 for all independent reflections (R_1 = 0.0371 was calculated for 3661 observed reflections with I > 2σ(I)). All the calculations were performed using SHELX2018 [28]. The CCDC 2034871 contains the supplementary crystallographic data for **8**. These data can be obtained free of charge via http://www.ccdc.cam.ac.uk/conts/retrieving.html (or from the CCDC, 12 Union Road, Cambridge, CB21EZ, UK; or deposit@ccdc.cam.ac.uk).

Computational details: All the calculations were conducted in the Gaussian09 program (rev. D01) [28]. The geometry optimization procedures were performed using standard criteria on displacements and forces. The DFT optimization were performed using the PBE0 functional [29,30] and the 6-311++G(d,p) basis set (ultrafine integration grids were used). The non-specific solvation was modelled using the self-consistent reaction field approach (PCM model, ε = 72). The influence of specific solvation on the geometry of **8** was accounted for by the optimization of a central molecule in clusters; two models were used: (1) the trimer of molecules from crystal of **8** with fixed coordinates and normalized X-H bond lengths for lateral molecules and (2) the shell of molecules from crystal of **8** with fixed coordinates and normalized X-H bond lengths. The Quantum theory of Atoms in Molecules surface integrals for the trimer were calculated using the AIMAll program [31]. The shell in the second model was generated using the criteria of at least one geometrical contact (within the sum of van der Waals radii plus 5 Å) between the surrounding molecules and the central molecule. The shell was described by the ONIOM approach (PBE0/6-311++G(d,p):PBE0/3-21G), and only the internal layer (the central molecule) was optimized. The Hessian calculations for all the optimized structures revealed their correspondence to energy minimums.

3. Results

3.1. o-Carboranyl-Cysteine Synthesis

The reaction conditions for the sulfa-Michael addition of thiophenols to methyl 2-acetamidoacrylate are well-studied [32]. It has been shown that reactions proceed in toluene or THF with catalytic quantity of the basic salt K_2CO_3 in the presence of solid-liquid phase-transfer catalyst. On the one hand, it was reasonable to apply conditions studied for thiophenols to the mercapto derivative of *o*-carborane; however, prolonged reaction with a base may cause of a side reaction due to the well-known property of *o*-carborane to undergo deboronation in the presence of bases, even mild ones, to yield *nido*-[7,9-$C_2B_9H_{12}$] [33–39]. The deboronation of *o*-$C_2B_{10}H_{12}$ proceeds fairly easily, whereas *m*-$C_2B_{10}H_{12}$, which was used for the synthesis of **6**, is much more stable under the same conditions. A detailed study of such differences has been presented [40]. On the other hand, more common work up of *o*-carboranyl thiols includes the conversion of the formed SH-derivative to the more stable triethylammonium [41,42] or trimethylammonium salt [27] **7** (Scheme 1). The usage of the trimethylammonium salt **7** let us to avoid the deprotonation stage during the reaction process to keep the *o*-carborane structure from degradation under the action of a base. The synthetic route developed for the preparation of the cysteine derivative of *o*-carborane conjugate with cysteine is outlined in Scheme 1.

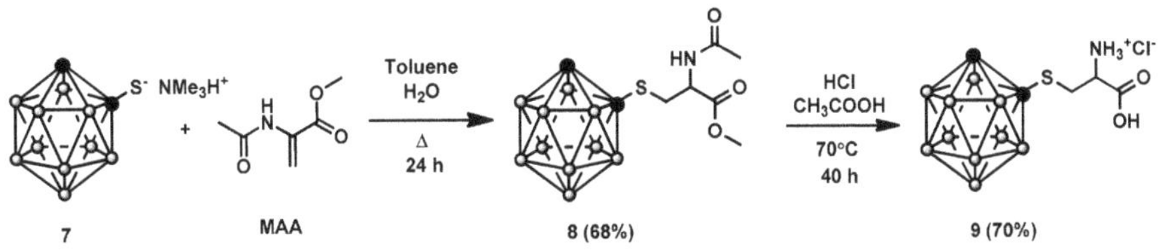

Scheme 1. Synthesis of *o*-carboranyl cysteine.

Compared to mercapto-*o*-carborane, *o*-carboranyl thiolate **7** lacks sufficient acidic hydrogen, which is necessary for the reaction to proceed. We found that reaction of **7** with methyl 2-acetamidoacrylate in a biphasic toluene-H_2O system under reflux for 24 h without base or any additional catalyst results in the formation of sulfa-Michael addition reaction product **8**.

The structure of **8** was confirmed by ^{1}H, ^{11}B, ^{13}C NMR, and IR spectroscopy, high-resolution mass spectrometry, and single-crystal X-ray diffraction study. The ^{1}H NMR spectrum of **8** in $CDCl_3$ shows two singlets at 2.06 and 3.83 due to the acetamide and the ester groups, a doublet at 6.17 ppm from the NH-group, a multiplet at 4.90 ppm attributed to the proton bonded to the α-carbon, two doublet of doublets at 3.51 and 3.18 ppm assigned to the diastereotopic methylene protons, and a broad singlet of carborane C-H group at 3.99 ppm. The ^{13}C-NMR spectrum contains signals of two carbonyl groups at 170.21 and 170.17 ppm., two cluster carbons at 73.9 and 67.9 ppm, two methyls of ester at 53.2 and acetamide at 23.1 ppm., as well as the CH and CH_2 groups at 51.2 and 39.4 ppm. The ^{11}B and $^{11}B\{^{1}H\}$ NMR spectra are in agreement with the C-mono-substituted o-carborane structure.

The solid-state structure of **8** was determined by single-crystal X-ray diffraction. The molecule of **8** is crystallized as the racemate in the centrosymmetric P-1 space group and contains a stereocenter at the C4 atom (Figure 2).

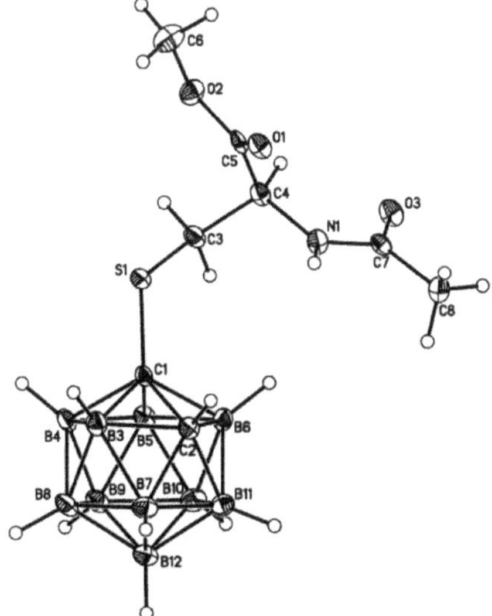

Figure 2. General view of the molecule **8** in crystal. Non-hydrogen atoms are given as probability ellipsoids of atomic displacements ($p = 0.5$).

While the main structural features of **8** are expected for this class of compounds (the C1-C2, S1-C1, and S1-C3 bond lengths equal 1.669(2), 1.791(1), and 1.826(1) Å, respectively; the sum of valence angles at the amide-type N1 atom equals 358.9°), the rotation of the substituent at the C1 atom with respect to the carborane cage can, however, hardly be rationalized by common intramolecular structural effects. For instance, the lone electron pairs of the S1 atom are nearly periplanar to the C3-H and C3-C4 bonds that contradicts the preferred geometry of expected LP(S)→σ* stereoelectronic interactions (Figure 3a). Indeed, the Cambridge Structural Database search reveals the predominance of staggered conformations of the C-S_{sp3}-C_{sp3}-C_{sp3} fragments (Figure 3b), whereas the corresponding torsion angle equals 118.1(2)° in **8**.

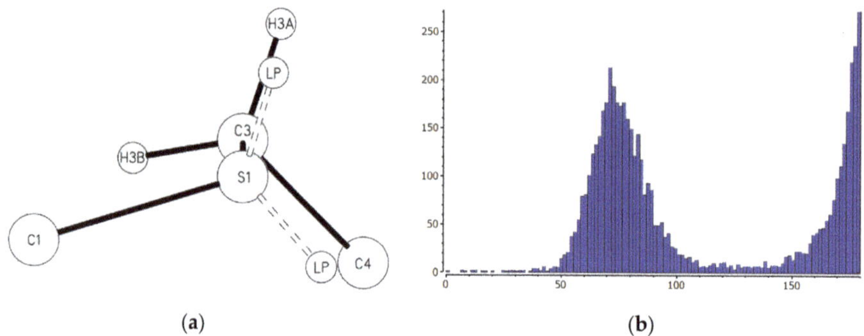

Figure 3. The conformation of the C1-S1-C3-C4 fragment in **8** (LP–positions of lone electronic pairs, (**a**)) and the distribution of corresponding torsion angles in the C-S_{sp3}-C_{sp3}-C_{sp3} fragments retrieved from the Cambridge Structural Database (**b**).

Based on the geometrical analysis of the crystal packing of **8**, it has been found that the substituent conformation could be stabilized by the environment effects. Indeed, there are several shortened intermolecular contacts formed by atoms of the C1 substituent which can be attributed to rather strong interactions – NH ... O H-bonds (N1 ... O1 2.933(2) Å, NHO 161.3° with normalized N-H bond length) and O ... π interactions (O1 ... O3 3.020(2) Å), both bounding molecules into infinite chains (Figure 4). The weak BH ... HC and CH ... O interactions are the only meaningful interactions between these chains.

In order to reveal the influence of environment effects on the conformation of **8**, the DFT calculations were additionally performed. Indeed, both the isolated molecule optimization and the optimization of **8** accounting for non-specific solvation effects (the SCRF-PCM model, relative dielectric permittivity of 72) produced structures being significantly different from those observed in the crystal: the root-mean-square deviations of the best overlap for non-hydrogen atoms are 0.495 and 0.446 Å, respectively. Surprisingly, the explicit DFT treatment of three neighboring molecules from a chain (see Figure 4) forming the mentioned shortened intramolecular contacts did not lead to any pronounced changes: the rmsd value for the central molecule in the calculated trimer equals 0.320 Å. Note that the total energy of mentioned N-H ... O H-bonds and O ... π interactions exceeds 24 kcal·mol^{-1} according to the QTAIM electron density analysis [43] carried out for the trimer. Our best result was achieved by the ONIOM calculation, which considers all neighboring molecules at the DFT level (the rmsd value equals to 0.168 Å, Figure 5). Thus, despite the relatively large strength of the H-bonds and O ... π interactions, the conformation of **8** in crystal depends heavily on the peculiarities of other, weaker intermolecular interactions such as BH ... HC and CH ... O.

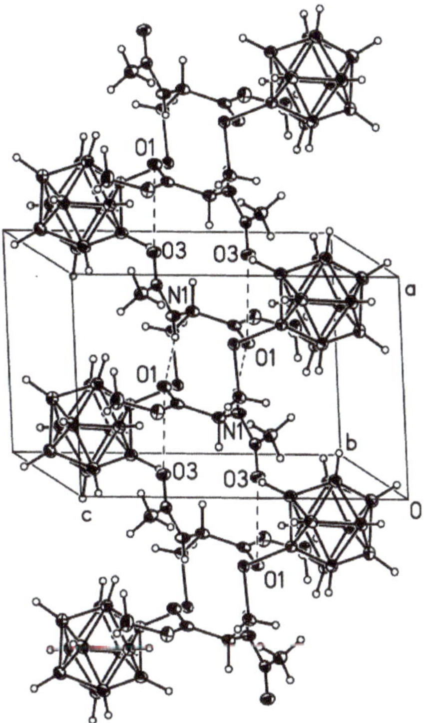

Figure 4. A fragment of the infinite chain formed in crystal of **8** along the *a* axis. Non-hydrogen atoms are given as probability ellipsoids of atomic displacements ($p = 0.5$).

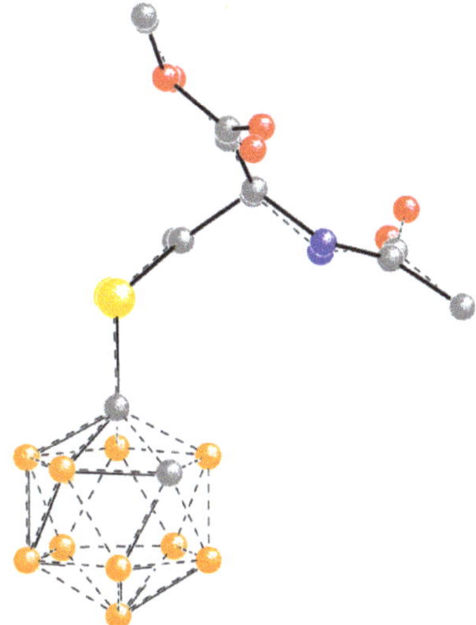

Figure 5. The best root-mean-square overlap for non-hydrogen atoms between crystal (solid lines) and ONIOM-modelled (dashed lines) conformations of **8**.

The treatment of **8** with a mixture of glacial acetic and hydrochloric acids under heating gave the title S-substituted cysteine **9** in the form of hydrochloride with a good yield (Scheme 1). The synthesized amino acid was characterized by ^{1}H, ^{11}B, ^{13}C NMR spectroscopy, IR spectroscopy, and high-resolution mass spectrometry. A singlet at 4.89 ppm corresponding to the C-H from the o-carborane was observed in the ^{1}H NMR; other chemical shifts agreeing with amino acid structure were also observed.

3.2. The Sulfa-Michel Addition Mechanism Investigation for o-Carboranyl Cysteine and Synthesis of Deuterium Labeled Compounds

The investigation of the reaction conditions for the synthesis of **8** revealed a crucial role of the choice of solvent. Thus, the formation of only an insignificant amount of **8** was observed when the reaction proceeded in homogenous systems EtOH-H_2O or THF-H_2O, whereas in absolute EtOH no product was detected at all. The best result was achieved when the toluene-H_2O system was used without any base. Since the initial salt **7** did not have an acid proton, as 1-mercapto-o-carborane has, this is why we assumed that α-proton comes into intermediate **8** from water. To gain some insight into the process, we carried out the "free of base" reaction with $^{2}H_2O$, which required strictly anhydrous conditions (Scheme 2).

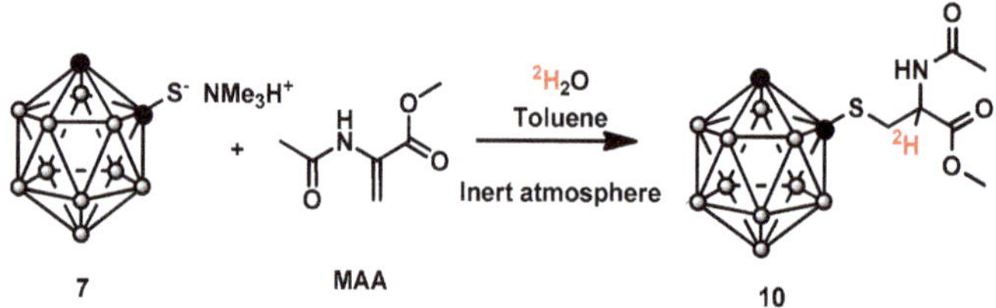

Scheme 2. Synthesis of the labeled with deuterium *o*-carboranyl conjugate.

We found that the two-phase system reaction proceeds in the way we proposed. Compound **10** with deuterium at the α-position of amino acid was isolated and characterized by NMR, IR spectroscopy, and mass spectrometry. The reaction time for the synthesis of **10** in the toluene-$^{2}H_2O$ system increased as compared with those in the toluene-H_2O system. This difference in reaction time may be attributed to the presence of a deuterium isotope effect. The yield of reaction, which was detected, remains over 65%. The comparison of the ^{1}H NMR and ^{13}C spectra of **8** and **10** is displayed below (Figure 6).

The ^{1}H NMR spectrum of **10** in $CDCl_3$ does not contain the multiplet at 4.90 ppm, which indicates the absence of a proton at the α-position of the amino acid, whereas in the ^{13}C-NMR spectrum the triplet due to the $C^{2}H$ group appears at 51.0 ppm, indicating the substitution of H for ^{2}H. In addition, the doublet of the NH group (6.17 ppm) and two doublets of doublets from the methylene CH_2 protons, which were detected in the ^{1}H NMR spectrum of **8**, collapsed to a singlet and two doublets in the spectrum of [α-^{2}H]carboranyl-cysteine **10**, respectively, due to the absence of an adjacent proton.

The subsequent acid hydrolysis of **10** resulted in the o-carboranyl-cysteine **11**, labeled at the α-position of the amino acid (Scheme 3).

The presence of ^{2}H and its position were determined by high-resolution mass spectrometry and ^{1}H NMR spectroscopy. The ^{1}H NMR spectrum showed the presence of an unlabeled compound in an amount of less than 10% (Figure 7).

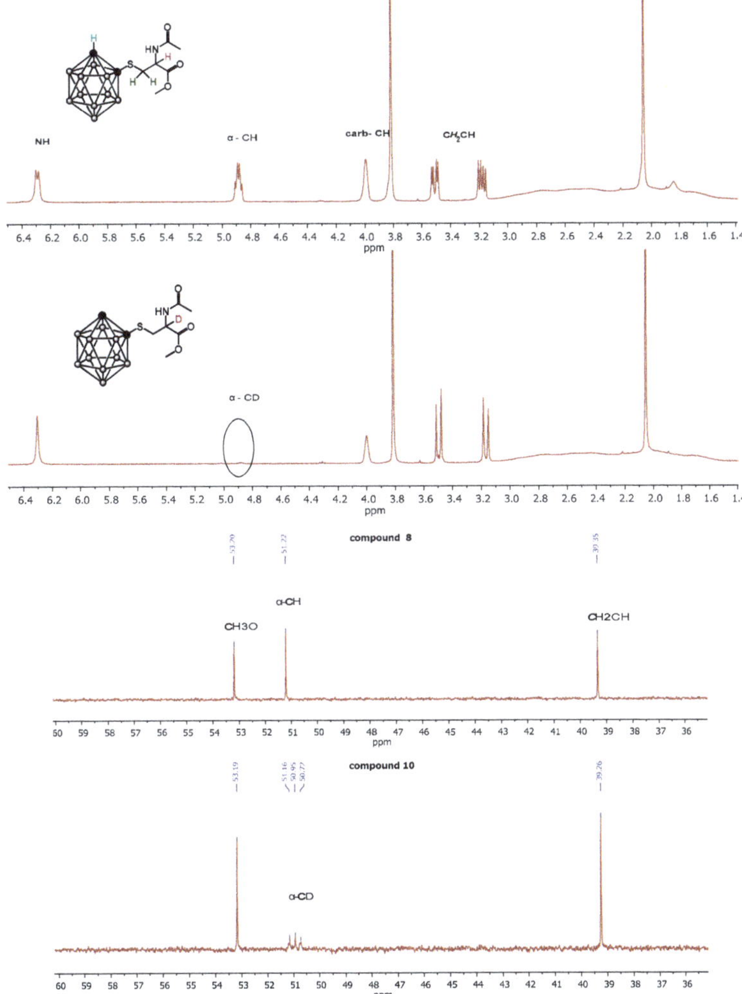

Figure 6. Comparison of ^{1}H NMR and fragments of the ^{13}C NMR spectra of **8** and **10** in $CDCl_3$.

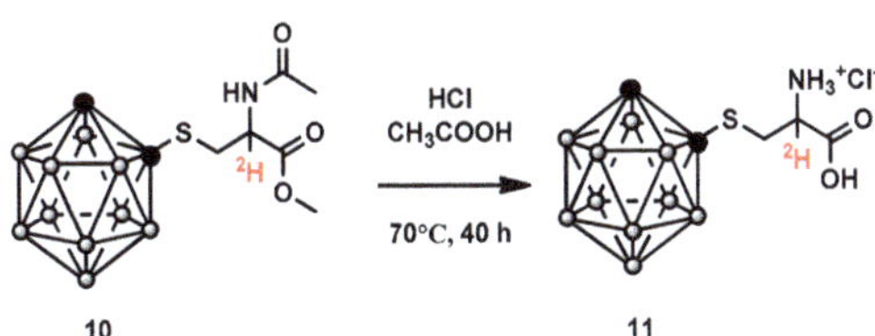

Scheme 3. *O*-carboranyl-DL-[α-^{2}H]-cysteine synthesis.

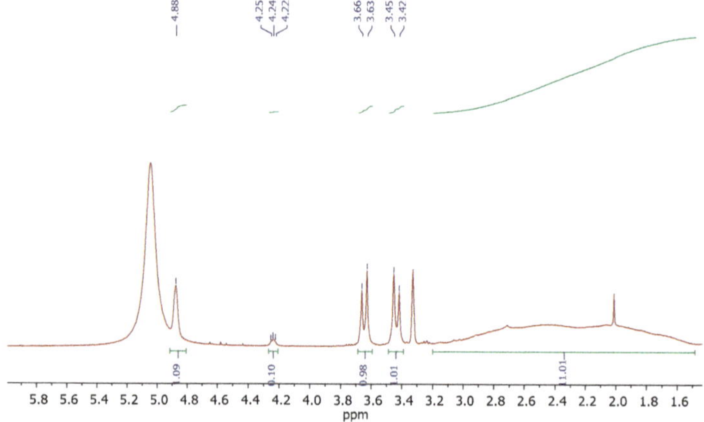

Figure 7. ^{1}H NMR spectrum of **11** in methanol-d_4.

The method proposed above can be considered as a preparative one for the synthesis of labeled o-carboranyl-DL-[α-^{2}H]-cysteine, which could be useful for study of the metabolism of o-carboranyl-DL-cysteine itself, as well as the metabolism of boron-containing proteins on its base as potential BNCT agents [44–46].

It was mentioned that the o-carborane system is sensitive to the presence of a base. To investigate the effect of water-soluble basic salt toward the reaction that proceeds in a two-phase system, we added K_2CO_3 to the reaction system. We found that the addition of a basic salt accelerates the reaction, which is complete in 8 h, but resulted in an only 17% yield of **8**, while the main product is *nido*-carborane derivatives, as found by ^{11}B NMR. The solvent change from H_2O to $^{2}H_2O$ along with the use of anhydrous K_2CO_3 and a Schlenk technique under an atmosphere of argon increases the reaction time from 8 h to 10 h due to the isotope effect, and the yield of product falls from 17% to 10%. Interestingly, the structure of the resulting product was found to be different from **8** and **10**. According to the NMR spectroscopy data, deuterium from $^{2}H_2O$ took up a place of the 1-CH-*o*-carborane proton, whereas proton appeared at the α-position of the amino acid (Scheme 4, Figure 8). Compound **12** was isolated and characterized, and its structure and composition were confirmed by ^{1}H, ^{11}B, ^{13}C NMR, and IR spectroscopy and high-resolution mass spectrometry.

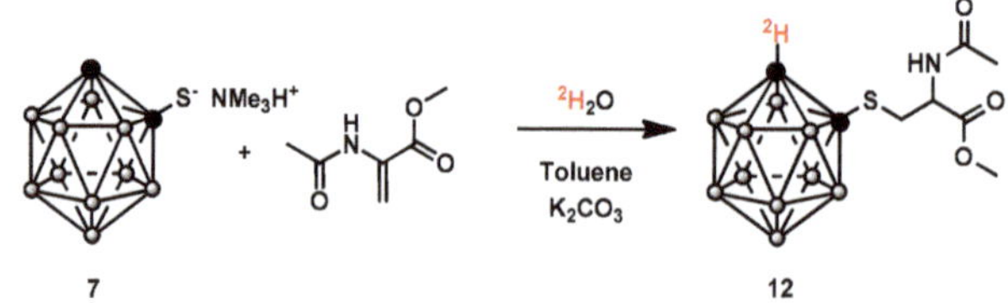

Scheme 4. The sulfa-Michael addition reaction in the presence of the basic salt.

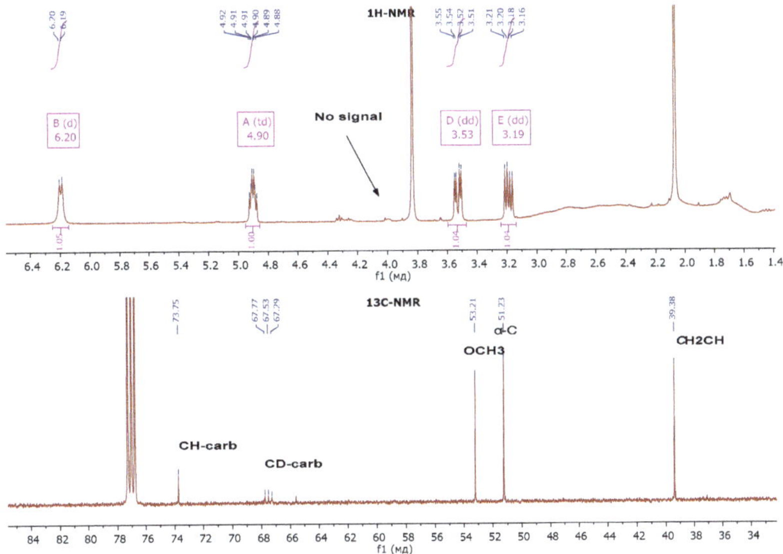

Figure 8. ^{1}H and a fragment of ^{13}C NMR spectra of **12** in $CDCl_3$.

4. Discussion

To summarize the obtained results, we assumed the mechanism of reaction proceeding (Scheme 5).

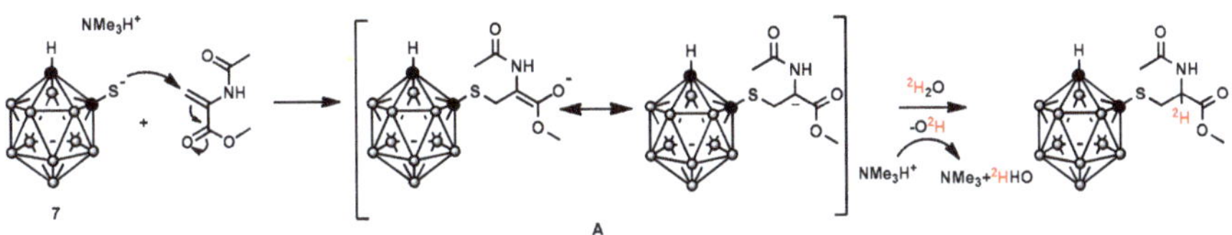

Scheme 5. Proposed mechanism of the reaction of trimethylammonium salt of 1-mercapto-*o*-carborane with methyl 2-acetamidoacrylate.

The reaction realizes according to a classical Michael addition reaction, where thiolate **7** acts as a nucleophile without additional deprotonation. In the first step, nucleophile reacts with the electrophilic alkene to form **A** in a conjugate addition reaction. In the next stage, the deuterium abstraction from solvent by the enolate **A** forms the final conjugate and a $^2HO^-$ anion from a water molecule. $^2HO^-$ anion, being a base, may cause a deboronation process, however its cooperation with a cation forms a water-soluble trimethylammonium hydroxide. When the reaction proceeds in the toluene-^2H_2O system, trimethylammonium hydroxide eliminates from the toluene medium and under the reaction conditions it decomposes in an aqueous medium with the formation of trimethylamine and water. Thus, the final stage process may be described as proton abstraction from cation that results in the deactivation of a base. The proposed mechanism is also supported by the fact that an increase in the reaction time does not have a significant effect on the yield of **8**. The reaction between **7** and methyl 2-acetamidoacrylate in EtOH does not give the desired product. According to the proposed mechanism, in this case the proton abstraction from solvent by the enolate **A** forms an EtO^- anion, which is not eliminated from the reaction system. The EtO^- anion being formed may undergo the Michael addition reaction, as well as **7** and/or deboronate *o*-carborane structure. The explanation above can be applied to a reaction in a system of two miscible liquids, such as THF-H_2O. The formed hydroxide anion remains in one system with the reactants to yield mainly a *nido*-carborane product.

5. Conclusions

Two possibilities of the sulfa-Michael addition reaction in the synthesis of *o*-carboranyl-DL-cysteine were investigated. The reaction proceeding between the trimethylammonium salt of 1-mercapto-*o*-carborane and methyl 2-acetamidoacrylate in the two-phase system, toluene-H_2O with base, as expected, demonstrates a low yield. Using the "free of base" method under the mild conditions in the two-phase system, the side processes were minimized and after the deprotection 1-HOOCCH(NH_2)CH_2S-1,2-$C_2B_{10}H_{11}$ was obtained in a good total yield. The developed "free of base" method was applied for the preparation of *o*-carboranyl-DL-cysteine labeled with deuterium at the α-position of amino acid using cheap and easily available ^2H_2O as a deuterium source. The obtained compounds can be considered as potential agents for the Boron Neutron Capture Therapy of cancer as well as for protein metabolism studies.

Supplementary Materials: The following are available online at http://www.mdpi.com/2073-4352/10/12/1133/s1.

Author Contributions: Synthesis and writing—original draft preparation, J.L.; synthesis, M.S.; NMR research analysis, I.K.; X-ray diffraction study, I.A.; supervision, V.B. and I.S. All authors have read and agreed to the published version of the manuscript.

Funding: This work was supported by the Russian Science Foundation (№ 19-72-30005).

Acknowledgments: The NMR spectroscopy studies and X-ray diffraction experiment were performed using equipment of the Center for Molecular Structure Studies at A.N. Nesmeyanov Institute of Organoelement Compounds operating with financial support of the Ministry of Science and Higher Education of the Russian Federation.

Conflicts of Interest: The authors declare no conflict of interest.

References

1. Siegel, R.L.; Miller, K.D.; Jemal, A. Cancer statistics. *CA Cancer J. Clin.* **2019**, *69*, 7–34. [CrossRef] [PubMed]
2. Black, P.M. Brain Tumors. *N. Engl. J. Med.* **1991**, *324*, 1471–1476. [CrossRef] [PubMed]
3. Shah, H.K.; Mehta, M.P. Radiation Therapy. In *High-Grade Gliomas. Current Clinical Oncology*; Barnett, G.H., Ed.; Humana Press: Totowa, NJ, USA, 2007; pp. 231–244. [CrossRef]
4. Afseth, J.; Neubeck, L.; Karatzias, T.; Grant, R. Holistic needs assessment in brain cancer patients: A systematic review of available tools. *Eur. J. Cancer Care* **2018**, *28*, e12931. [CrossRef]
5. Locher, G.L. Biological effects and therapeutic possibilities of neutrons. *Am. J. Roentgenol. Radium Ther.* **1936**, *36*, 1–13.
6. Tolpin, E.I.; Wellum, G.R.; Dohan, F.C., Jr.; Kornblith, P.R.; Zamenhof, R.G. Boron Neutron Capture Therapy of Cerebral Gliomas. *Oncology* **1975**, *32*, 223–246. [CrossRef] [PubMed]
7. Barth, R.F.; Zhang, Z.; Liu, T. A realistic appraisal of boron neutron capture therapy as a cancer treatment modality. *Cancer Commun.* **2018**, *38*, 36. [CrossRef] [PubMed]
8. Xuan, S.; Vicente, M.G.H. Recent Advances in Boron Delivery Agents for Boron Neutron Capture Therapy (BNCT). In *Boron-Based Compounds: Potential and Emerging Applications in Biomedicine*; Hey-Hawkins, E., Viñas, C., Eds.; John Wiley & Sons: Hoboken, NJ, USA, 2018; pp. 298–342.
9. Henriksson, R.; Capala, J.; Michanek, A.; Lindahl, S.-Å.; Salford, L.G.; Franzén, L.; Blomquist, E.; Westlin, J.-E.; Bergenheim, T.A. Boron Neutron Capture Therapy (BNCT) for Glioblastoma Multiforme: A Phase II Study Evaluating A Prolonged High-Dose of Boronophenylalanine (BPA). *Radiother. Oncol.* **2008**, *88*, 183–191. [CrossRef]
10. Kulvik, M.; Vähätalo, J.; Buchar, E.; Färkkilä, M.; Järviluoma, E.; Jääskeläinen, J.; Křiž, O.; Laakso, J.; Rasilainen, M.; Ruokonen, I.; et al. Clinical implementation of 4-dihydroxyborylphenylalanine synthesised by an asymmetric pathway. *Eur. J. Pharm. Sci.* **2003**, *18*, 155–163. [CrossRef]
11. Barth, R.F.; Coderre, J.F.; Vicente, M.G.H.; Blue, T.E. Boron Neutron Capture Therapy of Cancer: Current Status and Future Prospects. *Clin. Cancer Res.* **2005**, *11*, 3987–4002. [CrossRef]

12. Hu, K.; Yang, Z.; Zhang, L.; Xie, L.; Wang, L.; Xu, H.; Josephson, L.; Liang, S.H.; Zhang, M.-R. Boron agents for neutron capture therapy. *Coord. Chem. Rev.* **2020**, *405*, 213139. [CrossRef]
13. Kabalka, G.W.; Yao, M.-L. The synthesis and use of boronated amino acids for boron neutron capture therapy. *Anticancer Agents Med. Chem.* **2006**, *6*, 111–125. [CrossRef] [PubMed]
14. Hawthorne, M.F. The Role of Chemistry in the Development of Boron Neutron Capture Therapy of Cancer. *Angew. Chem. Int. Ed. Engl.* **1993**, *32*, 950–984. [CrossRef]
15. Sivaev, I.B.; Bregadze, V.I. Polyhedral Boranes for Medical Applications: Current Status and Perspectives. *Eur. J. Inorg. Chem.* **2009**, 1433–1450. [CrossRef]
16. Grimes, R.N. *Carboranes*, 3rd ed.; Academic Press: New York, NY, USA; Elsevier: Amsterdam, The Netherlands, 2016.
17. Stogniy, M.Y.; Zakharova, M.V.; Sivaev, I.B.; Godovikov, I.A.; Chizov, A.O.; Bregadze, V.I. Synthesis of new carborane-based amino acids. *Polyhedron* **2013**, *55*, 117–120. [CrossRef]
18. Leukart, O.; Caviezel, M.; Eberle, A.; Escher, E.; Tun-Kyi, A.; Schwyzer, R. L-o-Carboranylalanine, a Boron Analogue of Phenylalanine. *Helv. Chim. Acta* **1976**, *59*, 2184–2187. [CrossRef]
19. Gruzdev, D.A.; Levit, G.L.; Olshevskaya, V.A.; Krasnov, V.P. Synthesis of ortho-Carboranyl Derivatives of (S)-Asparagine and (S)-Glutamine. *Russ. J. Org. Chem.* **2017**, *5*, 769–776. [CrossRef]
20. Prashar, J.K.; Moore, D.E. Synthesis of Carboranyl Phenylalanine for Potential Use in Neutron Capture Therapy of Melanoma. *J. Chem. Soc. Perkin Trans. 1* **1993**, 1051–1053. [CrossRef]
21. Gruzdev, D.A.; Ustinov, V.O.; Levit, G.L.; Ol'shevskaya, V.A.; Krasnov, V.P. Synthesis of meta-Carboranyl-(S)-homocysteine Sulfoxide. *Russ. J. Org. Chem.* **2018**, *54*, 1579–1582. [CrossRef]
22. He, T.; Misuraca, J.C.; Musah, R.A. "Carboranyl-Cysteine"-Synthesis, Structure and Self-Assembly Behavior of a Novel α-Amino Acid. *Sci. Rep.* **2017**, *7*, 16995. [CrossRef]
23. He, T.; Musah, R.A. Evaluation of the Potential of 2-Amino-3-(1,7-dicarba-closododecaboranyl-1-thio)propanoic Acid as a Boron Neutron Capture Therapy Agent. *ACS Omega* **2019**, *4*, 3820–3826. [CrossRef]
24. He, T.; Chittur, S.V.; Musah, R.A. Impact on Glioblastoma U87 Cell Gene Expression of a Carborane Cluster bearing Amino Acid: Implications for Carborane Toxicity in Mammalian Cells. *ACS Chem. Neurosci.* **2019**, *10*, 1524–1534. [CrossRef] [PubMed]
25. Vinas, C.; Benakki, R.; Teixidor, F.; Casabo, J. Dimethoxyethane as a Solvent for the Synthesis of C-Monosubstituted o-Carborane Derivatives. *Inorg. Chem.* **1995**, *34*, 3844–3845. [CrossRef]
26. Plešek, J.; Heřmanek, S. Syntheses and properties of substituted icosahedral carborane thiols. *Collect. Czech. Chem. Commun.* **1981**, *46*, 687–692. [CrossRef]
27. Stogniy, M.Y.; Erokhina, S.A.; Druzina, A.A.; Sivaev, I.B.; Bregadze, V.I. Synthesis of novel carboranyl azides and "click" reactions thereof. *J. Organomet. Chem.* **2019**, *904*, 121007. [CrossRef]
28. Frisch, M.J.; Trucks, G.W.; Schlegel, H.B.; Scuseria, G.E.; Robb, M.A.; Cheeseman, J.R.; Scalmani, G.; Barone, V.; Petersson, G.A.; Nakatsuji, H.; et al. *Gaussian 09, Revision, D.01*; Gaussian, Inc.: Wallingford, CT, USA, 2016.
29. Perdew, J.; Ernzerhof, M.; Burke, K. Rationale for mixing exact exchange with density functional approximations. *J. Chem. Phys.* **1996**, *105*, 9982–9985. [CrossRef]
30. Carlo, A.; Barone, V. Toward reliable density functional methods without adjustable parameters: The PBE0 model. *J. Chem. Phys.* **1999**, *110*, 6158–6170. [CrossRef]
31. Keith, T.A. *TK Gristmill Software*; AIMAll (Version 19.10.12): Overland Park, KS, USA, 2019.
32. Cossec, B.; Cosnier, F.; Burgart, M. Methyl Mercapturate Synthesis: An Efficient, Convenient and Simple Method. *Molecules* **2008**, *13*, 2394–2407. [CrossRef]
33. Davidson, M.G.; Fox, M.A.; Hibbert, T.G.; Howard, J.A.K.; Mackinnon, A.; Neretin, I.S.; Wade, K. Deboronation of orthocarborane by an iminophosphorane: Crystal structures of the novel carborane adduct nido-$C_2B_{10}H_{12}$·HNP(NMe_2)$_3$ and the borenium salt [(Me_2N)$_3$PNHBNP(NMe_2)$_3$]$_2O_2^+$ ($C_2B_9H_{12}^-$)$_2$. *Chem. Commun.* **1999**, 1649–1650. [CrossRef]
34. Svantesson, E.; Pettersson, J.; Olin, Å.; Markides, K.E. A kinetic study of the self-degradation of *o*-carboranylalanine to *nido*-carboranylalanine in solution. *Acta Chem. Scand.* **1999**, *53*, 731–736. [CrossRef]
35. Taoda, Y.; Sawabe, T.; Endo, Y.; Yamaguchi, K.; Fujii, S.; Kagechika, H. Identification of an intermediate in the deboronation of *ortho*-carborane: An adduct of *ortho*-carborane with two nucleophiles on one boron atom. *Chem. Commun.* **2008**, 2049–2051. [CrossRef]

36. Kononov, L.O.; Orlova, A.V.; Zinin, A.I.; Kimel, B.G.; Sivaev, I.B.; Bregadze, V.I. Conjugates of polyhedral boron compounds with carbohydrates. 2. Unexpected easy *closo*- to *nido*-transformation of a carborane–carbohydrate conjugate in neutral aqueous solution. *J. Organomet. Chem.* **2005**, *690*, 2769–2774. [CrossRef]
37. Likhosherstov, L.M.; Novikova, O.S.; Chizhov, A.O.; Sivaev, I.B.; Bregadze, V.I. Conjugates of polyhedral boron compounds with carbohydrates 8. Synthesis and properties of *nido-ortho*-carborane glyco conjugates containing one to three β-lactosylamine residues. *Russ. Chem. Bull.* **2011**, *60*, 2359–2364. [CrossRef]
38. Núñez, R.; Teixidor, F.; Kivekäs, R.; Sillanpää, R.; Viñas, C. Influence of the solvent and R groups on the structure of (carboranyl)R_2PI_2 compounds in solution. Crystal structure of the first iodophosphonium salt incorporating the anion $[7,8\text{-nido-}C_2B_9H_{10}]^-$. *Dalton Trans.* **2008**, 1471–1480. [CrossRef]
39. Teixidor, F.; Viñas, C.; Mar Abad, M.; Nuñez, R.; Sillanpäa, R. Procedure for the degradation of 1,2-$(PR_2)_2$-1,2-dicarba-*closo*-dodecaborane(12) and 1-(PR_2)-2-R′-1,2-dicarba-*closo*-dodecaborane(12). *J. Organomet. Chem.* **1995**, *503*, 193–203. [CrossRef]
40. Poater, J.; Viñas, C.; Bennour, I.; Escayola, S.; Solà, M.; Teixidor, F. Too Persistent to Give up: Aromaticity in Boron Clusters Survives Radical Structural Changes. *J. Am. Chem. Soc.* **2020**, *142*. [CrossRef] [PubMed]
41. Boyd, L.A.; Clegg, W.; Copley, R.C.B.; Davidson, M.G.; Fox, M.A.; Hibbert, T.G.; Howard, J.A.; Mackinnon, K.A.; Peace, R.J.; Wade, K. Exo-π-bonding to an *ortho*-carborane hypercarbon atom: Systematic icosahedral cage distortions reflected in the structures of the fluoro-, hydroxy- and amino-carboranes, 1-X-2-Ph-1,2-$C_2B_{10}H_{10}$ (X = F, OH or NH_2) and related anions. *Dalton Trans.* **2004**, 2786–2799. [CrossRef] [PubMed]
42. Stogniy, M.Y.; Sivaev, I.B.; Petrovskii, P.V.; Bregadze, V.I. Synthesis of monosubstituted functional derivatives of carboranes from1-mercapto-*ortho*-carborane: 1-HOOC(CH_2)nS-1,2-$C_2B_{10}H_{11}$ and $[7\text{-HOOC}(CH_2)\text{nS-}7,8\text{-}C_2B_9H_{11}]^-$ (n = 1–4). *Dalton Trans.* **2010**, *39*, 1817–1822. [CrossRef]
43. Romanova, A.; Lyssenko, K.; Ananyev, I. Estimations of energy of noncovalent bonding from integrals over interatomic zero-flux surfaces: Correlation trends and beyond. *J. Comput. Chem.* **2018**, *39*, 1607–1616. [CrossRef]
44. Mutlib, A.E. Application of Stable Isotope-Labeled Compounds in Metabolism and in Metabolism-Mediated Toxicity Studies. *Chem. Res. Toxicol.* **2008**, *21*, 1672–1689. [CrossRef]
45. Wilkinson, D.J. Historical and contemporary stable isotope tracer approaches to studying mammalian protein metabolism. *Mass Spectrom. Rev.* **2018**, *37*, 57–80. [CrossRef]
46. Pająk, M.; Pałka, K.; Winnicka, E.; Kańska, M. The chemo- enzymatic synthesis of labeled l-amino acids and some of their derivatives. *J. Radioanal. Nucl. Chem.* **2018**, *317*, 643–666. [CrossRef] [PubMed]

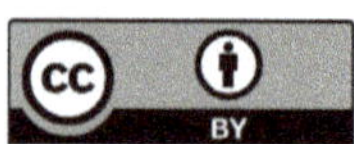

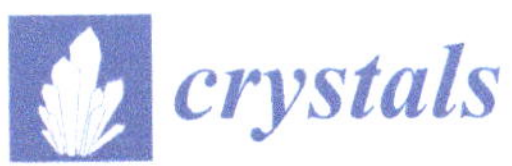 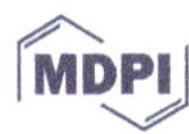

Article

Reactions of Experimentally Known *Closo*-$C_2B_8H_{10}$ with Bases. A Computational Study

Josef Holub [1], Jindřich Fanfrlík [2], Michael L. McKee [3] and Drahomír Hnyk [1,*]

1 Institute of Inorganic Chemistry of the Czech Academy of Sciences, CZ-250 68 Husinec-Řež, Czech Republic; holub@iic.cas.cz
2 Institute of Organic Chemistry and Biochemistry of the Czech Academy of Sciences, CZ-166 10 Praha 6, Czech Republic; jindrich.fanfrlik@marge.uochb.cas.cz
3 Department of Chemistry and Biochemistry, Auburn University, Auburn, AL 36849, USA; mckeeml@auburn.edu
* Correspondence: hnyk@iic.cas.cz

Received: 19 August 2020; Accepted: 29 September 2020; Published: 3 October 2020

Abstract: On the basis of the direct transformations of *closo*-1,2-$C_2B_8H_{10}$ with $OH^{(-)}$ and NH_3 to *arachno*-1,6,9-$OC_2B_8H_{13}{}^{(-)}$ and *arachno*-1,6,9-$NC_2B_8H_{13}$, respectively, which were experimentally observed, the DFT computational protocol was used to examine the corresponding reaction pathways. This work is thus a computational attempt to describe the formations of 11-vertex *arachno* clusters that are formally derived from the hypothetical *closo*-$B_{13}H_{13}{}^{(2-)}$. Moreover, such a protocol successfully described the formation of *arachno*-4,5-$C_2B_6H_{11}{}^{(-)}$ as the very final product of the first reaction. Analogous experimental transformations of *closo*-1,6-$C_2B_8H_{10}$ and *closo*-1,10-$C_2B_8H_{10}$, although attempted, were not successful. However, their transformations were explored through computations.

Keywords: carboranes; DFT; reaction pathways

1. Introduction

Polyhedral borane and heteroborane clusters are known for the presence of delocalized electron-deficient bonding [1,2] and characterized by forming three-center, two-electron (3c-2e) bonds. This bonding is quite different from organic chemistry that is dominated by classical two-center two-electron (2c-2e) bonds. The trigonal faces of boranes and carboranes are assembled to create three-dimensional shapes such as icosahedron and bicapped-square antiprism [2] appearing in *closo* systems. The preparation and subsequent reactivity of these clusters have been extensively studied by experiments [1,2]. In particular, the 12-vertex icosahedral *closo* clusters have been one of the main targets. In contrast to well-understood reaction mechanisms in organic chemistry, those in boron cluster chemistry can be very complex because there are very small energy differences between many intermediates and transition states. On that basis, the reaction of boron hydrides may involve many competing pathways [3]. For that reason, relatively little progress has so far been made in the understanding of the reaction mechanisms of boron hydrides and carboranes of various molecular shapes [4–6]. To our knowledge, the reaction pathways associated with ten-vertex *closo* carboranes, for instance *closo*-1,2-$C_2B_8H_{10}$ (see Scheme 1), have not yet been explored.

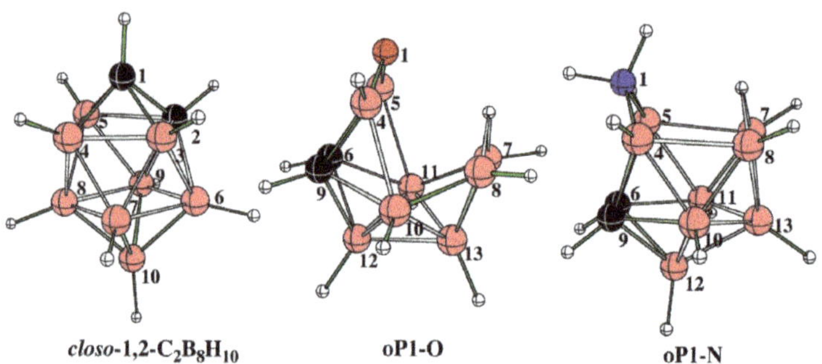

Scheme 1. Molecular diagrams of *closo*-1,2-$C_2B_8H_{10}$, *arachno*-1,6,9-$OC_2B_8H_{13}{}^{(-)}$ (**oP1-O**), and *arachno*-1,6,9-$NC_2B_8H_{13}$ (**oP1-N**) and the corresponding atomic numberings.

The $C_2B_8H_{10}$ molecular shape of a bicapped-square antiprism exists in seven positional isomers, only three of which (1,2-, 1,6- and 1,10-isomers) are known experimentally [2]. The most stable one is the 1,10-isomer and the least stable one is the 2,3-isomer [7]. The 1,6-isomer has recently been examined experimentally [8]. In addition, a new synthetic pathway for the preparation of the 1,2-isomer has also been outlined, including some mechanistic considerations [9]. Mutual isomerizations of all the possible *closo*-$C_2B_8H_{10}$ have been studied computationally [10]. As to the observed reactivity of the 1,2-isomer, its direct *closo* to *arachno* transformations have been experimentally observed [11,12], with the resulting *arachno* structural motif being based on the hypothetical *closo*-$B_{13}H_{13}{}^{(2-)}$ as also seen from the corresponding atomic numberings (see also Scheme 1) [13]. Since no computational work has been reported in the area of the reactions of 10-vertex *closo* carboranes, we have undertaken a computational study of the experimentally known isomers of *closo*-$C_2B_8H_{10}$ with the Lewis bases $OH^{(-)}$ and NH_3. Both bases are hard in terms of the HSAB theory of acids and bases [14] with $OH^{(-)}$ being harder than NH_3 on the HSAB scale.

2. Methods

All of the stationary points in the reactions of *closo*-1,2-, 1,6-, and 1,10-$C_2B_8H_{10}$ with $OH^{(-)}$ were optimized and frequencies were calculated at the SMD(water) [15,16]/B3LYP/6-311+G(2d,p) level, a model chemistry well-established for this class of materials [4–6]. The entries in Table 1 for B3LYP/6-311+G(2d,p) are single-point energies at SMD(water)/B3LYP/6-311+G(2d,p)-optimized geometries. The reactions of the same carborane with neutral NH_3 were optimized at the B3LYP/6-311+G(2d,p) level without taking solvation effects into account, which is quite reasonable for neutral species. Moreover, unlike the investigation of organic reaction mechanisms where the bonding is 2c–2e and bond-breaking reaction steps can cause the wave function to become unstable with respect to symmetry-breaking, in the investigation of electron deficient reactions, the bonding scheme fluidly changes between different patterns of multi-center bonding. While dynamic electron correlation is important (and described by the B3LYP approach used in this study), non-dynamic (i.e., static) electron correlation (caused by near degeneracy effects) is not important. All of the transition states were relaxed in terms of the application of the intrinsic reaction coordinate (IRC) approach at the SMD(water)/B3LYP/6-31+G(d) level for the reactions with $OH^{(-)}$ and at the B3LYP/6-31G(d) level for the reactions with NH_3, and the structures obtained are very similar to those obtained with the 6-311+G(2d,p) basis set. In order to check the possible influence of dispersion corrections, the wB97XD/6-311+G(2d,p), model chemistry was also employed for some stationary points. All the computations were performed using Gaussian09, in which the above model chemistries and basis sets are incorporated [17].

Table 1. Solvation free energies (kcal·mol^{-1}), and free energies relative to the appropriate reference. The small "o" refers to ortho (1,2-) $C_2B_8H_{10}$. The capital letters "**A**", "**B**", "**C**", etc. and "TS#" are related to individual intermediates and transition states, respectively. If there were two conformations possible, two letters are used to differentiate between them (e.g., **oG/G′-O, oK/K′-O** and **oM/M′-O**). The capital "**-O**" and "**-N**" distinguish between the reactions of $OH^{(-)}$ and NH_3, respectively. Wherever the intermediate is relatively stable (and already isolated or possibly trappable), "**P1**", "**P2**", "**P3**", etc. are used instead of "**A**", "**B**", "**C**".

Notation	ΔG (solv) [1]	ΔG (aq,298K) [2]	Notation	ΔG (solv) [1]	ΔG (aq,298K) [2]
	$C_2B_8H_{10}$ + OH $^{(-)}$ [3]			**$C_2B_8H_{10}$ + NH_3 [4]**	
$OH^{(-)}$	−94.76		NH_3	−3.67	
H_2O	−2.05		H_2BNH_2	−1.24	
H_2BOH	−3.82		**oTS1-N**	−4.70	32.1
OBOH	−14.65		**oA-N**	−11.06	15.8
$B(OH)_3$			**oTS2-N**	−0.43	50.3
oTS1-O	−53.74	27.2	**oP1-N**	−3.75	−1.3
oA-O	−46.19	2.0	**oTS3-N**	−0.64	43.8
oTS2O	−42.58	10.0	**oB-N**	−0.39	23.8
oB-O	−44.80	1.8	**oTS4-N**	−1.46	32.8
oTS3-O	−39.89	14.5	**oC-N**	−0.34	24.4
oP1-O	−40.16	−18.4	**oTS5-N**	−0.01	32.3
4,5-$C_2B_6H_{11}{}^{(-)}$	−39.67	−50.7	**oD-N**	0.27	31.2
oC-O	−41.59	−18.2	**oTS6-N**	0.81	39.5
oTS4-O	−45.21	18.5	**P2-N**	−3.48	7.3
oD-O	−47.70	−2.2	**oTS7-N**	−1.01	38.3
oTS5-O	−48.36	9.1	**oE-N**	−0.55	29.5
oE-O	−47.59	0.0	**oTS8-N**	0.49	36.4
oTS6-O	−47.61	0.2	**oP3-N**	−3.20	11.1
oF-O	−45.17	−1.2	**oTS9-N**	−3.06	32.1
oTS7-O	−43.15	8.8	**oF-N**	−3.30	29.7
oP2-O	−45.07	−18.8	**oTS10-N**	−6.51	29.8
oTS8-O	−58.47	6.2	**oG-N**	−2.08	25.1
oG-O	−63.94	1.6	**oTS11-N**	−2.74	35.0
oG′-O	−63.85	1.6	**oH-N**	−2.77	26.5
oTS9-O	−50.19	7.9	**oTS12-N**	−2.22	39.1
oH-O	−53.32	4.6	**oI-N**	−1.85	32.0
oTS10-O	−51.94	5.7	**oTS13-N**	−1.97	32.8
oI-O	−66.84	0.1	**oP4-N**	−2.27	−5.5
oJ-O	−60.59	−1.1			
oTS11-O	−58.96	−1.5			
oK-O	−48.64	−27.9			
oK′-O	−44.34	−26.8			
oTS12-O	−45.37	-19.5			
oL-O	−51.68	−26.9			
oM-O	−56.47	−28.4			
oM′-O	−53.96	−29.2			
oTS13-O	−58.13	−4.2			
4,5-$C_2B_6H_{11}{}^{(-)}$	−39.43	−41.7			

[1] Solvation free energies (the energy difference between B3LYP/6-311+G(2d,p) and SMD/B3LYP/6-311+G(2d,p) at 298.15 K (kcal·mol^{-1}). [2] Relative free energies in kcal·mol^{-1} (where the references are 1,2-$C_2B_8H_{10}$+$OH^{(-)}$ for $OH^{(-)}$ and 1,2-$C_2B_8H_{10}$+NH_3 for NH_3 reactions). The ΔG(aq,298K) and ΔG(solv) for 1,2-$C_2B_8H_{10}$ are 0.0 kcal·mol^{-1} and −0.5 kcal·mol^{-1}, respectively. The solvation free energy of H_2O is taken from the experiment (−2.05 kcal·mol^{-1}). In some cases, H_2NBH_2 is added for mass balance. In the formation of $C_2B_6H_{11}{}^{(-)}$, the comparison is made with respect to 1,2-$C_2B_8H_{10}$ + $OH^{(-)}$+3H_2O. [3] Geometry optimizations and frequencies calculated at the SMD(water)/B3LYP/6-311+G(2d,p) level of theory. [4] Geometry optimizations and frequencies calculated at the B3LYP/6-311+G(2d,p) level of theory.

3. Results and Discussion

3.1. The Reaction with Hydroxides

The first part of the reaction of 1,2-$C_2B_8H_{10}$ with $OH^{(-)}$ is a quite straightforward process. This experimentally verified reaction, with the **oP1-O** final product, arachno-1,6,9-$OC_2B_8H_{13}^{(-)}$ (Scheme 1), proceeds through three transition states (TSs) and two intermediates, with the latter still bearing $OH^{(-)}$ (see Figure 1). The B-H-B bridge is a result of H migration to the B(7)–B(8) position in the final step of this reaction cascade. However, when one molecule of H_2O is added to **oP1-O**, the cluster further degrades and through seven TSs an intermediate **oI-O** is obtained, which is prone to further degradation, when another water molecule is added to the O–B–O–H chain through two hydrogen bonds. This initiation results, via selective degradation of B(3,6)-cage atoms, in the formation of arachno-$C_2B_6H_{11}^{(-)}$ through a number of TSs and intermediates, this arachno system being also isolated experimentally (see Figures 1 and 2 and Table 1) [18]. Note that the first barrier associated with **oTS1-O** was also examined with wB97XD/6-311+G(2d,p) and no significant difference from the B3LYP/6-311+G(2d,p) value was found, i.e., 24.9 kcal·mol^{-1} vs. 27.2 kcal·mol^{-1} as seen from Table 1. The potential energy surface attributed to the reaction of 1,6-$C_2B_8H_{10}$ + $OH^{(-)}$ was rather difficult to follow. Since this reaction was not observed experimentally, we moved this computational effort to Supplementary Materials (see Figures S1 and S2). The geometrical shape of the final product **mP3-O** bears a slight resemblance to the nido-11 vertex geometry, but not with the open pentagonal belt because the $OH^{(-)}$ group migrates through the entire process without any indication of the insertion of oxygen into the cage boron atoms (see Figure S1). The mechanism of the reaction of the 1,10 isomer with $OH^{(-)}$, also not observed experimentally, is even more complex. Interestingly, the final product (**pP1-O**, see Figures S3 and S4) of the latter reaction is of the same molecular shape, i.e., with a B–O–B bridge, as in the case of the reaction of 1,2-$C_2B_8H_{10}$ with $OH^{(-)}$ (**oP1-O**), but it originates through five TSs instead of three.

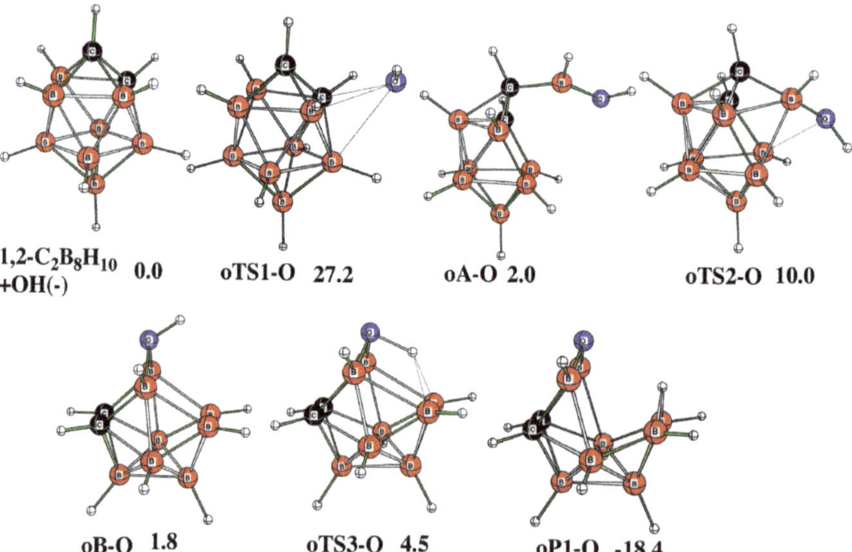

Figure 1. *Cont.*

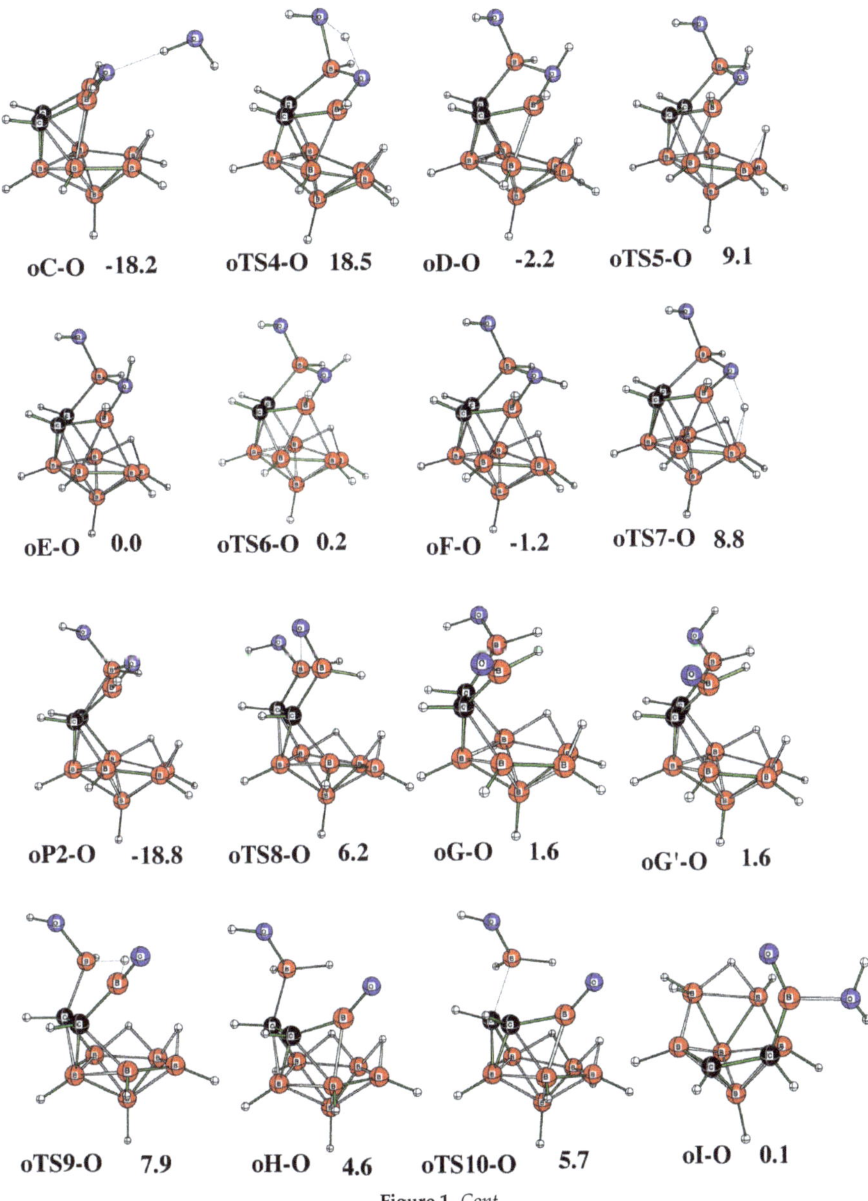

Figure 1. *Cont.*

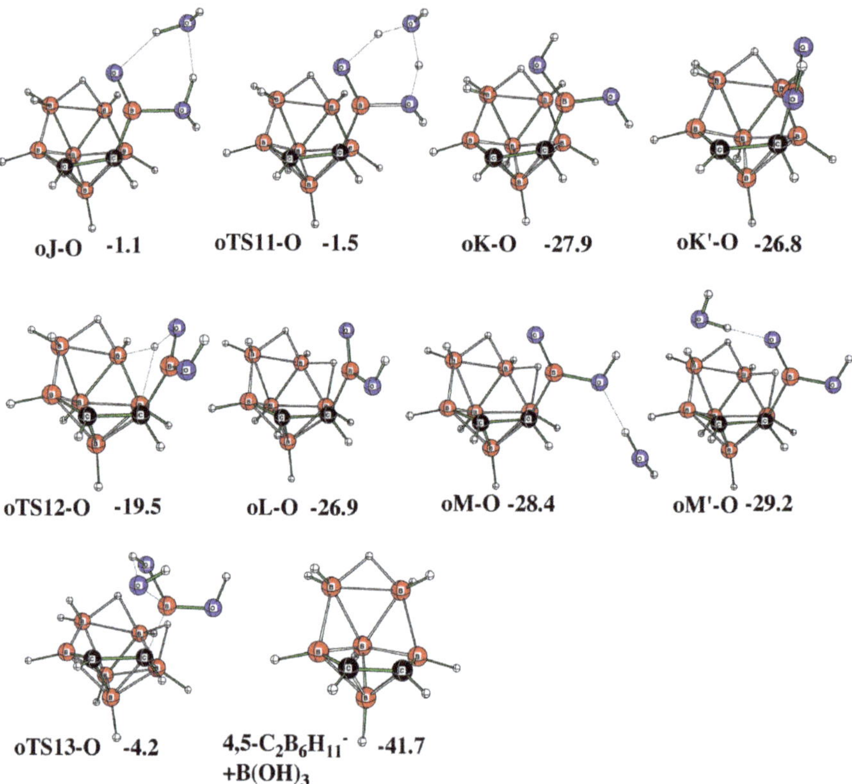

Figure 1. Individual stationary points as determined in the reaction pathway of the reaction of *closo*-1,2-$C_2B_8H_{10}$ with $OH^{(-)}$.

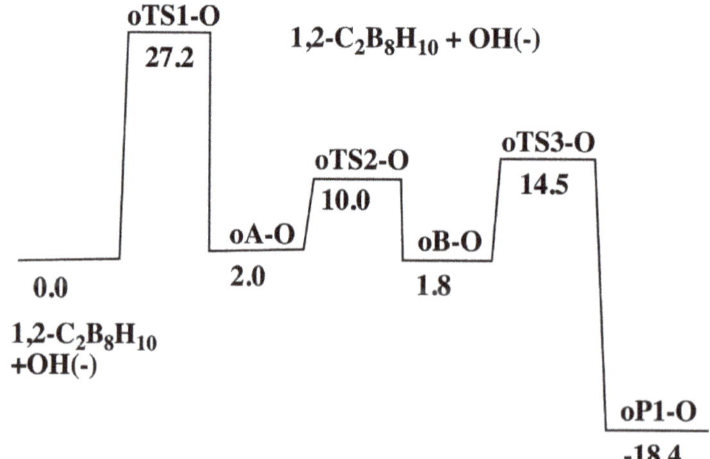

Figure 2. *Cont.*

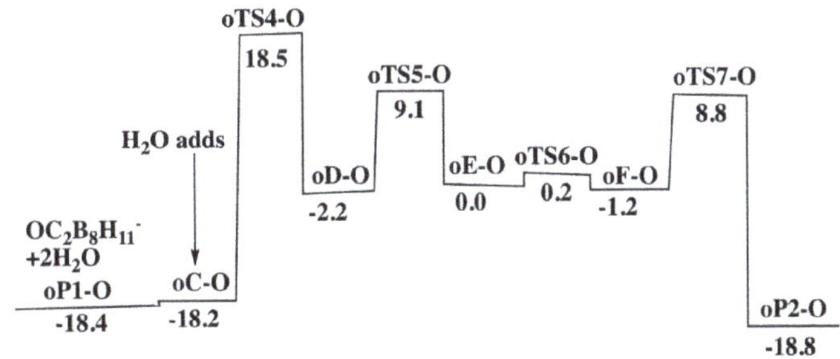

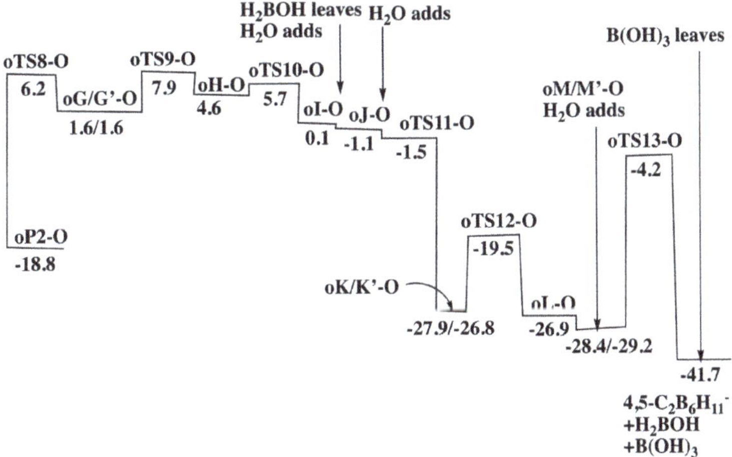

Figure 2. Relative free energies (kcal·mol^{-1}) of the individual stationary points on the Potential Energy Surface (PES) of the reaction of *closo*-1,2-$C_2B_8H_{10}$ with $OH^{(-)}$ (see Table 1 and Methods for details).

3.2. The Reaction with Amines

The reaction of *closo*-1,2-$C_2B_8H_{10}$ with NH_3 has been experimentally known to provide *arachno*-1,6,9-$NC_2B_8H_{13}$ (Scheme 1) [11,17]. The initiation of this reaction is based on the attack of NH_3 on the most positive boron within the cage, i.e., B(3), which forms a triangle with both C vertices. The highest free energy barrier (50.3 kcal·mol^{-1}) is **TS2-N**, through which the NH_3 group becomes NH_2 in the 1,6,9 isomer denoted as **oP1-N** in the reaction pathway (see Figures 3 and 4 and Table 1). However, this experimentally known part of the entire reaction (see above) occurs without any large intervening barriers and, consequently, the **oP1-N** isomer is obtained through two transition states and one intermediate. The same is apparently true for various amines of the R_1R_2NH type [19]. This reaction proceeds through a series of intermediate steps to the known 1,8,11-isomer (**oP2-N**), experimentally available by another procedure [20]. To our knowledge, there is no experimental evidence of the conversion of **oP2-N** to **oP1-N**, although this process is computed to be exothermic ($\Delta G = -8.6$ kcal·mol^{-1}). Note that the experimentally detected *arachno*-1,6,9-$NC_2B_8H_{13}$ originates under less exothermic conditions than its oxygen analog. In analogy with the reaction of 1,2-$C_2B_8H_{10}$ with $OH^{(-)}$, we also examined the first barrier using wB97XD/6-311+G(2d,p) and again no significant difference from the B3LYP/6-311+G(2d,p) value was computed, i.e., 28.3 kcal·mol^{-1} vs. 32.1 kcal·mol^{-1} as provided by Table 1. When the 1,6,9-isomer (**oP1-N**) was examined computationally in terms of searching for another TS, i.e., **oTS7-N**, it isomerizes to a new isomer, **oP3-N**, through two TSs and one intermediate, **oE-N**, with the C–C bond remains intact as judged by a separation of 1.565 Å. When the

C–C separation was increased, another TS and intermediate, i.e., **oTS9-N** and **oF-N**, respectively, were located with much longer C ... C separations of 2.409 and 2.774 Å, respectively. This significant geometrical change initiates a continuation of the reaction through other four subsequent TSs to the next known isomer, i.e., **oP4-N**. The reaction of the 1,6-isomers (see Figures S5 and S6) was a result of the simultaneous initial attack of NH_3 on B(3) and C(6); the N atom forms a cap above the B(2)B(3)C(6) triangle in the transition state with a free energy barrier of 34.6 kcal·mol^{-1}. The second free energy barrier was even higher, 52.0 kcal·mol^{-1} and might account for the fact that this reaction does not occur experimentally. Interestingly, when the common product of the reactions of *closo*-1,2-$C_2B_8H_{10}$ and *closo*-1,6-$C_2B_8H_{10}$ with NH_3, i.e., **oP4-N**, is reached (see also Figure S5), both reactions proceed in the same way and *closo*-$C_2B_7H_9$ is obtained, where the two carbon atoms are separated from each other. Basically, there are five isomers of *closo*-$C_2B_7H_9$. The isomerization barrier between the most stable C_{2v} (C ... C separation) and the third most stable C_1 (C–C bond) forms is quite high (36 kcal·mol^{-1}). The high barrier is not unusual as isomerizations involving the C–C bond in carboranes often have rather high barriers. This type of *closo/closo* isomerization can also be described [21] in a more detailed way in terms of the consecutive double-Diamond-Square-Diamond (DSD) mechanism [10,22]. These two *closo* isomers have already been discussed by Schleyer [7] favoring the C_{2v}-symmetrical 4,5-isomer as well.

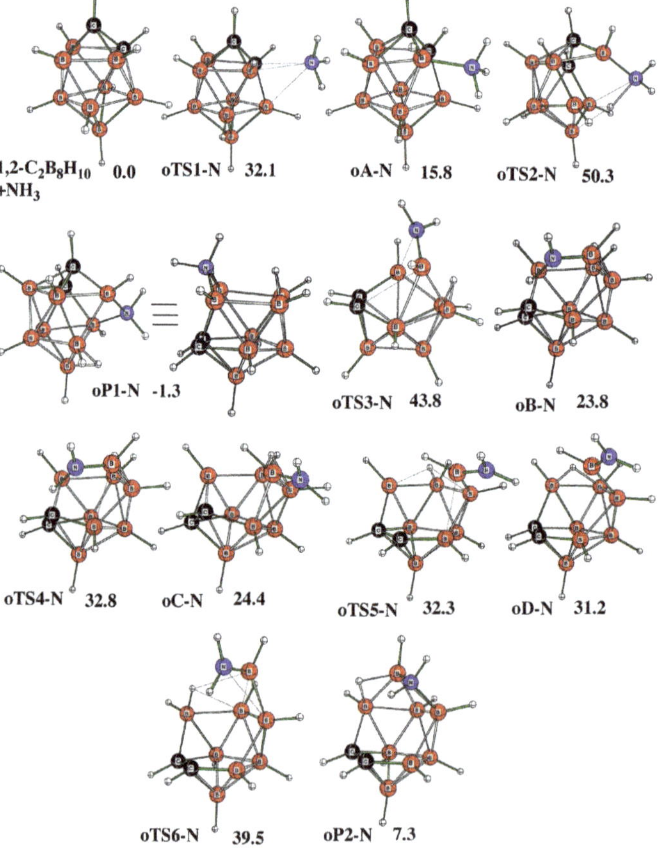

Figure 3. *Cont.*

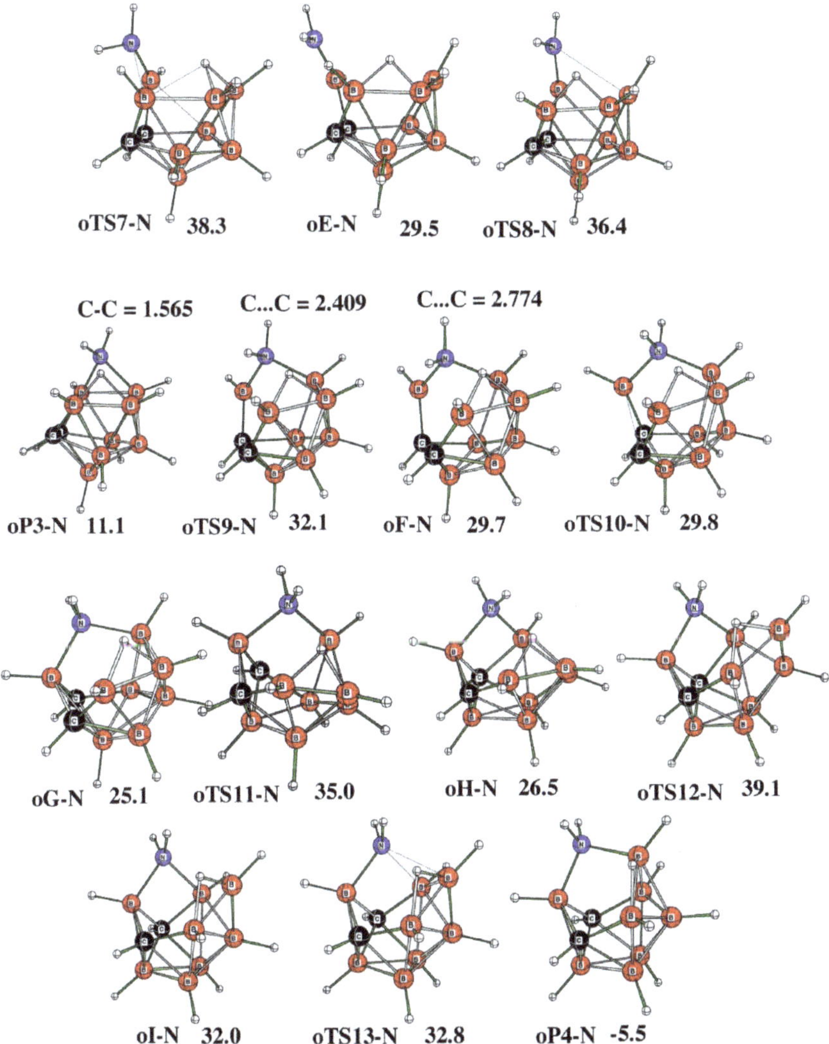

Figure 3. Individual stationary points on the PES of the reaction of *closo*-1,2-C_2B8H_{10} with NH_3.

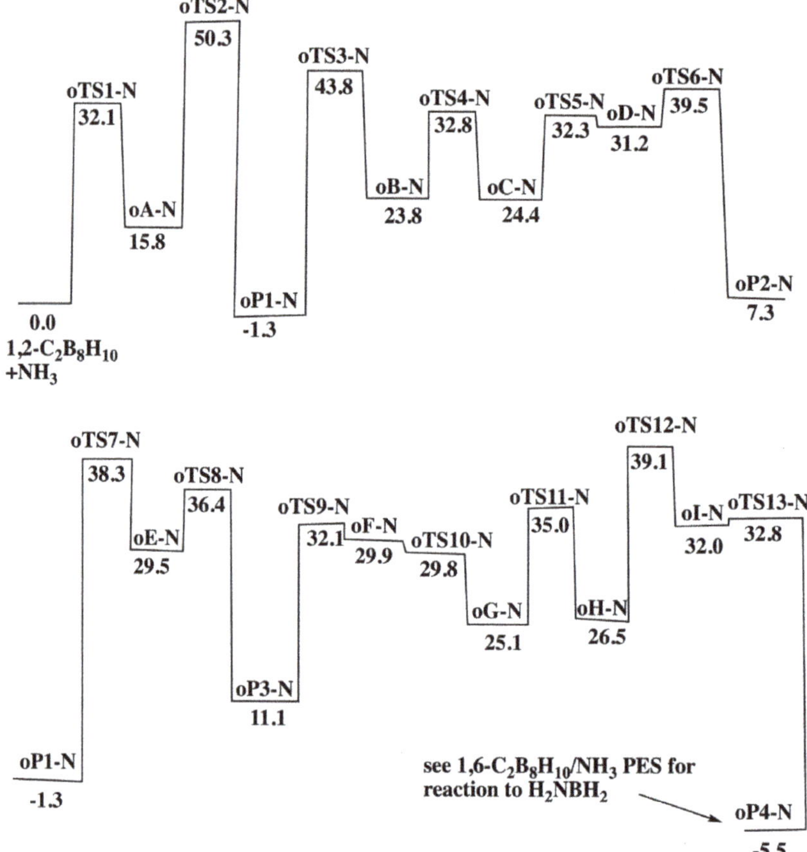

Figure 4. Relative free energies (kcal·mol^{-1}) of the individual stationary points on the PES of the reaction of *closo*-1,2-$C_2B_8H_{10}$ with NH_3 (see Table 1 and Methods for details).

The reaction of the 1,10 isomer with NH_3 is rather complex and proceeds through a cascade of TSs. The initial attack of NH_3 simultaneously takes place at the boron atoms of both CB_4 hemispheres (**pTS1-N**) with an initial free energy barrier of more than 60 kcal·mol^{-1} and *closo*-$C_2B_7H_9$ originating as the final product in the endothermic reaction, which is entirely the same as above (see Figures S7 and S8). The experimental reaction of neither the 1,6- nor the 1,10-isomer of $C_2B_8H_{10}$ with NH_3 have been successfully carried out.

4. Conclusions

The reaction pathways of the experimentally known reactions of *closo*-1,2-$C_2B_8H_{10}$ with both $OH^{(-)}$ and NH_3 were computed using the DFT protocol. The final predicted products from the extensive search of the potential energy surfaces correspond to the same products detected experimentally. Both the *closo*-1,6-$C_2B_8H_{10}$ and the *closo*-1,10-$C_2B_8H_{10}$ isomers were allowed to react with the $OH^{(-)}$ and NH_3 bases, without any defined products being observed. Finally, this work represents a computational attempt to study the debor reaction, in contrast to the debor principle [23] (the successive elimination of vertices), where boron vertices are removed in the course of the reaction as illustrated by obtaining *arachno*-$C_2B_6H_{11}{}^{(-)}$ as the very final product from the reaction of *closo*-1,2-$C_2B_8H_{10}$ with $OH^{(-)}$.

Supplementary Materials: The following are available online at http://www.mdpi.com/2073-4352/10/10/896/s1: Figure S1: Individual stationary points as detected in the reaction pathway of the reaction of *closo*-1,6-$C_2B_8H_{10}$ with $OH^{(-)}$, Figure S2: Relative free energies (kcal·mol^{-1}) of the individual stationary points on the PES of the reaction of *closo*-1,6-$C_2B_8H_{10}$ with $OH^{(-)}$, Figure S3: Individual stationary points as detected in the reaction pathway of the reaction of *closo*-1,10-$C_2B_8H_{10}$ with $OH^{(-)}$, Figure S4: Relative free energies (kcal·mol^{-1}) of the individual stationary points on the PES of the reaction of *closo*-1,10-$C_2B_8H_{10}$ with $OH^{(-)}$, Figure S5: Individual stationary points as detected in the reaction pathway of the reaction of *closo*-1,6-$C_2B_8H_{10}$ with NH_3, Figure S6: Relative free energies (kcal·mol^{-1}) of the individual stationary points on the PES of the reaction of *closo*-1,6-$C_2B_8H_{10}$ with NH_3, Figure S7: Individual stationary points as detected in the reaction pathway of the reaction of 1,10-$C_2B_8H_{10}$ with NH_3, Figure S8: Relative free energies (kcal·mol^{-1}) of the individual stationary points on the PES of the reaction of *closo*-1,10-$C_2B_8H_{10}$ with NH_3, Table S1: Number of imaginary frequencies, zero-point energies (kcal·mol^{-1}), heat capacity correction (kcal·mol^{-1}), entropies (cal.mol^{-1}·K^{-1}), solvation free energies (kcal·mol^{-1}), and free energies relative to the appropriate reference. Small o, m, or p refer to ortho (1,2-), meta (1,6-), or para (1,10-)$C_2B_8H_{10}$, respectively. Capital letters "A", "B", "C", etc. or "TS#" are related to individual intermediates or transition states, respectively. If there were two conformations possible, two letters are used to discern them (e.g., oG/G′-O, oK/K′-O, or oM/M′-O). Capital "-O" or "-N" distinguish between the reactions of OH(-) or NH3, respectively. In cases where the intermediate is relatively stable (and already isolated or possibly trappable), "P1", "P2", "P3", etc. is used instead of "A", "B", "C". Table S2: Cartesian coordinates of all species in Table S1

Author Contributions: Computations, M.L.M., J.F., and D.H.; synthesis, J.H. All authors have read and agreed to the published version of the manuscript.

Funding: We thank the Czech Science Foundation for financial support (project no. 19-17156S). MLM thanks Auburn University for access to the HOPPER computer.

Conflicts of Interest: The authors declare no conflict of interest.

References

1. Hnyk, D.; Wann, D.A. Boron: The Fifth Element. In *Challenges and Advances in Computational Chemistry and Physics*; Hnyk, D., McKee, M., Eds.; Springer: Dordrecht, The Netherlands, 2016; Volume 20, pp. 17–48.
2. Grimes, R.N. *Carboranes*, 3rd ed.; Academic Press: Cambridge, MA, USA, 2016.
3. McKee, M.L. Boron: The Fifth Element. In *Challenges and Advances in Computational Chemistry and Physics*; Hnyk, D., McKee, M., Eds.; Springer: Dordrecht, The Netherlands, 2016; Volume 20, pp. 121–138.
4. McKay, D.; Macgregor, S.A.; Welch, A.J. Isomerisation of *nido*-$[C_2B_{10}H_{12}]^{2-}$ Dianions: Unprecedented Rearrangements and New Structural Motifs in Carborane Cluster Chemistry. *Chem. Sci.* **2015**, *6*, 3117–3128. [CrossRef] [PubMed]
5. Shameena, O.; Pathak, B.; Jemmis, E.D. Theoretical Study of the Reaction of $B_{20}H_{16}$ with MeCN: *Closo/Closo* to *Closo/Nido* Conversion. *Inorg. Chem.* **2008**, *47*, 4375–4382. [CrossRef] [PubMed]
6. Štíbr, B.; Holub, J.; Bakardjiev, M.; Lane, P.D.; McKee, M.L.; Wann, D.A.; Hnyk, D. Unusual Cage Rearrangements in 10-Vertex *nido*-5,6-Dicarbaborane Derivatives: An Interplay between Theory and Experiment. *Inorg. Chem.* **2017**, *56*, 852–860. [CrossRef] [PubMed]
7. Schleyer, P.V.R.; Najafian, K. Stability and Three-Dimensional Aromaticity of closo-Monocarbaborane Anions, $CB_{n-1}H_n^-$, and *closo*-Dicarboranes, $C_2B_{n-2}H_n$. *Inorg. Chem.* **1998**, *37*, 3454–3457. [CrossRef] [PubMed]
8. Bakardjiev, M.; Štíbr, B.; Holub, J.; Padělková, Z.; Růžička, A. Simple Synthesis, Halogenation, and Rearrangement of *closo*-1,6-$C_2B_8H_{10}$. *Organometallics* **2015**, *34*, 450–454. [CrossRef]
9. Tok, O.L.; Bakardjiev, M.; Štíbr, B.; Hnyk, D.; Holub, J.; Padělková, Z.; Růžička, A. Click Dehydrogenation of Carbon-Substituted *nido*-5,6-C_2B8H_{12} Carboranes: A General Route to *closo*-1,2-$C_2B_8H_{10}$ Derivatives. *Inorg. Chem.* **2016**, *55*, 8839–8843. [CrossRef] [PubMed]
10. Gimarc, B.M.; Ott, J.J. Isomerization of Carboranes $C_2B_6H_{18}$, $C_2B_8H_{10}$ and $C_2B_9H_{11}$ by the Diamond-Square-Diamond Rearrangement. *J. Am. Chem. Soc.* **1987**, *109*, 1388–1392. [CrossRef]
11. Janoušek, Z.; Fusek, J.; Štíbr, B. The First Example of a Direct *closo* to *arachno* Cluster Expansion Reaction in Boron Cluster Chemistry. *J. Chem. Soc. Dalton Trans.* **1992**, 2649–2650. [CrossRef]
12. Hnyk, D.; Holub, J. Handles for the Dicarbadodecaborane Basket Based on [*arachno*-4,5-C_2B_8H13]$^-$: Oxygen. *Dalton Trans.* **2006**, 2620–2622. [CrossRef] [PubMed]
13. Schleyer, P.V.R.; Najafian, K.; Mebel, A.M. The Large *closo*-Borane Dianions, $B_nH_n^{2-}$ (n = 13–17) Are Aromatic, Why Are They Unknown? *Inorg. Chem.* **1998**, *37*, 6765–6772. [CrossRef] [PubMed]

14. For Example, Fleming, I. *Frontier Orbitals and Organic Chemical Reactions;* John Wiley and Sons: Chichester, Sussex, UK, 1976.
15. Marenich, A.V.; Cramer, C.J.; Truhlar, D.G. Universal Solvation Model Based on Solute Electron Density and on a Continuum Model of the Solvent Defined by the Bulk Dielectric Constant and Atomic Surface Tensions. *J. Phys. Chem. B* **2009**, *113*, 6378–6396. [CrossRef] [PubMed]
16. Marenich, A.V.; Cramer, C.J.; Truhlar, D.G. Performance of SM6, SM8, and SMD on the SAMPL1 test set for the prediction of small-molecule solvation free energies. *J. Phys. Chem. B* **2009**, *113*, 4538–4543. [CrossRef] [PubMed]
17. Frisch, M.J.; Trucks, G.W.; Schlegel, H.B.; Scuseria, G.E.; Robb, M.A.; Cheeseman, J.R.; Scalmani, G.; Barone, V.; Mennucci, B.; Petersson, G.A.; et al. *Gaussian 09, Revision, D.01;* Gaussian, Inc.: Wallingford, CT, USA, 2009.
18. Jelínek, T.; Štíbr, B.; Heřmánek, S.; Plešek, J. A New Eight-Vertex arachno-Dicarbaborane anion, $[4,5\text{-}C_2B_6H_{11}]^-$. *J. Chem. Soc. Chem. Commun.* **1989**, 804–805. [CrossRef]
19. Janoušek, Z.; Dostál, R.; Macháček, J.; Hnyk, D.; Štíbr, B. The First Member of the Eleven-Vertex Azadicarbaborane Series, 1,6,9-$NC_2B_8H_{13}$ and its N-alkyl Derivatives. *Dalton Trans.* **2006**, 4664–4671. [CrossRef] [PubMed]
20. Plešek, J.; Štíbr, B.; Hnyk, D.; Jelínek, T.; Heřmánek, S.; Kennedy, J.D.; Hofmann, M.; Schleyer, P.V.R. Dicarbaheteroborane Chemistry. Representatives of Two Eleven-Vertex Dicarbaazaundecaborane Families: *Nido*-10,7,8-NC_2B_8H11, Its N-Substituted Derivatives, and *arachno*-1,8,11-$NC_2B_8H_{13}$. *Inorg. Chem.* **1998**, *37*, 3902–3909. [CrossRef] [PubMed]
21. Ceulemans, A.; Goijens, G.; Nguyen, M.T. $C_2B_7H_9$: Snapshots of a Rearranging Carborane. *J. Am. Chem. Soc.* **1994**, *116*, 9395–9396. [CrossRef]
22. Lipscomb, W.N. Framework Rearrangement in Boranes and Carboranes. *Science* **1966**, *153*, 373–378. [CrossRef] [PubMed]
23. Wade, K. Structural and Bonding Patterns in Cluster Chemistry. *Adv. Inorg. Chem. Radiochem.* **1976**, *18*, 1–66.

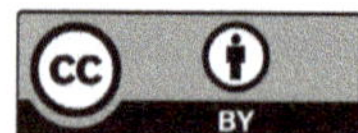

MDPI
St. Alban-Anlage 66
4052 Basel
Switzerland
Tel. +41 61 683 77 34
Fax +41 61 302 89 18
www.mdpi.com

Crystals Editorial Office
E-mail: crystals@mdpi.com
www.mdpi.com/journal/crystals

www.ingramcontent.com/pod-product-compliance
Lightning Source LLC
LaVergne TN
LVHW070623170726
843515LV00004B/167

* 9 7 8 3 0 3 6 5 3 6 1 9 4 *